Intra-Abdominal Hypertension

CORE CRITICAL CARE

Series Editor

Dr Alain Vuylsteke
Papworth Hospital
Cambridge, UK

Assistant Editor

Jo-anne Fowles
Papworth Hospital
Cambridge, UK

Other titles in the series

Delirium in Critical Care
Valerie Page and E. Wesley Ely
ISBN 9780521132534

Forthcoming titles in the series

Clinical Information Systems in Critical Care
Cecily Morrison, Matthew R. Jones and Julie Bracken
ISBN 9780521156745

Renal Replacement Therapy in Critical Care
Patrick Honoré and Oliver Joannes-Boyau
ISBN 9780521145404

Intra-Abdominal Hypertension

MANU MALBRAIN, MD, PHD

Director of ICU and High Care Burn Unit,
Ziekenhuis Netwerk Antwerpen (ZNA) Stuivenberg, Antwerp.
He is an ESICM Chris Stoutenbeek Award winner and the
Founding President of The World Society of the Abdominal
Compartment Syndrome (WSACS).

JAN DE WAELE, MD, PHD

Senior Lecturer at Ghent University and intensivist
at Ghent University Hospital, Ghent.
He is President of the WSACS (2013–2015).

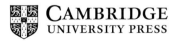

CAMBRIDGE
UNIVERSITY PRESS

CAMBRIDGE
UNIVERSITY PRESS

University Printing House, Cambridge CB2 8BS, United Kingdom

Published in the United States of America by Cambridge University Press, New York

Cambridge University Press is part of the University of Cambridge.

It furthers the University's mission by disseminating knowledge in the pursuit of education, learning and research at the highest international levels of excellence.

www.cambridge.org
Information on this title: www.cambridge.org/9780521149396

First published 2013

Printed by CPI Group (UK) Ltd, Croydon CR0 4YY

A catalogue record for this publication is available from the British Library

Library of Congress Cataloging in Publication data
Malbrain, Manu, 1965–
Intra-abdominal hypertension / Manu Malbrain, Jan De Waele.
 p. ; cm. – (Core critical care)
Includes bibliographical references.
ISBN 978-0-521-14939-6 (pbk.)
I. De Waele, Jan II. Title. III. Series: Core critical care.
[DNLM: 1. Intra-Abdominal Hypertension. WI 900]
RC691
616.1′3–dc23

                                        2013005145

ISBN 978-0-521-14939-6 Paperback

Additional resources for this publication at www.cambridge.org/malbrain

CONTENTS

CONTRIBUTORS

Definitions (Section 1)
MICHAEL L. CHEATHAM Department of Surgical
Education, Orlando Regional Medical Center, Orlando,
FL, USA

Principles of IAP Measurement (Section 1), Specific
Treatments (Section 5)
BART L. DE KEULENAER Department of Intensive Care,
Fremantle Hospital, WA, Australia

Decreased Abdominal Compliance (Section 2), Increased
Abdominal Content (Section 2), Central Nervous System
(Section 4), Renal System (Section 4), Improvement of
Abdominal Wall Compliance (Section 5), Correction of
Capillary Leak (Section 5)
INNEKE DE LAET Department of Intensive Care, Ziekenhuis
Netwerk Antwerpen, ZNA Stuivenberg, Antwerpen,
Belgium

Capillary Leak and Fluid Resuscitation (Section 2)
MICHAEL FRANCIS DITILLO AND LEWIS J. KAPLAN Department
of Surgery, Yale University School of Medicine, New Haven,
CT, USA

Children (Section 3)

J. CHIAKA EJIKE AND DONALD C. MOORES Department of Pediatric Critical Care Medicine, Loma Linda University, CA, USA

Burns (Section 3)

JUN ODA Department of Emergency and Critical Care Medicine, Tokyo Medical University Hospital, Tokyo, Japan

Obesity (Section 3)

HADLEY HERBERT, THERESE DUANE AND

RAO IVATURY Department of Surgery, Virginia Commonwealth University, Richmond, Virginia , USA

Pancreatitis (Section 3)

ARI LEPPANIEMI Department of Surgery, Meilahti hospital, University of Helsinki, Finland

Renal System (Section 4)

ERIC HOSTE Department of Intensive Care, University Hospital, Ghent, Belgium

How to Define Gastrointestinal Failure (Section 4)

ANNIKA REINTAM BLASER Department of Intensive Care, Tartu University Hospital, Tartu, Estonia

ABBREVIATIONS

ACCP	American College of Chest Physicians
ACS	abdominal compartment syndrome
AKI	acute kidney injury
APP	abdominal perfusion pressure
BMI	body mass index
C-abd	compliance abdominal wall
CAPD	chronic ambulatory peritoneal dialysis
CNAP	continuous negative abdominal pressure
CVP	central venous pressure
E-abd	elastance abdominal wall
EVLW	extravascular lung water
FG	filtration gradient
GEDV	global end-diastolic volume
GFP	glomerular filtration pressure
GID	gastrointestinal dysfunction
GIF	gastrointestinal failure
GIPS	global increased permeability syndrome
IAH	intra-abdominal hypertension
IAP	intra-abdominal pressure
IAPee	intra-abdominal pressure at the end of expiration

IAPei	intra-abdominal pressure at the end of inspiration
IAV	intra-abdominal volume
ICP	intracranial pressure
ICU	Intensive Care Unit
IGP	intragastric pressure
IVP	intravesicular pressure
LVEDV	left ventricular end-diastolic volume
MAP	mean arterial pressure
MODS	multiple organ dysfunction syndrome
MOF	multi-organ failure
NEXAP	negative extra-abdominal pressure
OCT	octreotide
PAOP	pulmonary arterial occlusion pressure
PCD	percutaneous drainage
PEEP	positive end expiratory pressure
PPV	pulse pressure variation
PTP	proximal tubular pressure
P/V	pressure–volume
Pv0	baseline pressure, measured without addition of volume
RRT	renal replacement therapy
SCCM	Society of Critical Care Medicine
SIRS	systemic inflammatory response syndrome
SOFA	sequential organ failure assessment
SVV	stroke volume variation
TAC	temporary abdominal closure
WSACS	World Society of the Abdominal Compartment Syndrome

FOREWORD

It is a pleasure to write the preface for this book in the
Core Critical Care series, entitled Intra-abdominal
Hypertension.

This book brings together in one volume all the clinician
needs to know about the physiology of intra-abdominal
pressure (IAP) in health and in disease. This knowledge is
crucial for the successful treatment of the critically ill, whether
medical or surgical, young or old. Intra-abdominal
hypertension (IAH) and the more sinister sequel, abdominal
compartment syndrome (ACS), have been known for at least
two centuries. We now understand that they are frequent
causes of increased morbidity and mortality in many of our ICU
patients. More importantly, we now know that they are
correctable causes, easily diagnosed and effectively treated,
only if the clinician is aware of the condition and pursues its
recognition.

Drs Malbrain and De Waele, as past President and
President-elect, respectively, of the World Society of Abdominal
Compartment Syndrome (WSACS), are leaders in this field. The
Society is a multispecialty, multinational and multitalented
association of individuals sharing a common goal – fostering
education and promoting awareness of IAH and ACS.

Both authors are renowned investigators and educators. In this book they have assembled what is truly important. The book provides readers with an easily accessible and readily digestible fund of knowledge that will, undoubtedly, translate into many saved lives. It is a useful bedside reference for all physicians, nurses and other members of the multidisciplinary team working in the ICU.

It is a personal privilege to be associated with the WSACS and this important work. I hope the reader studies it well and often, for he or she may savour the benefits of gained knowledge in grateful smiles from patients and their families.

Rao R. Ivatury MD, FACS
President
WSACS

Understanding intra-abdominal hypertension: what to worry about?

Chapter 1

What is intra-abdominal pressure?

Introduction

Awareness of the physiological importance of intra-abdominal pressure (IAP) has increased over the past 20 years.

It is important to understand the structure of the abdominal wall and its compliance (C-abd) to comprehend IAP fully, and how it relates to the content of the abdomen and thus intra-abdominal volume (IAV). IAP is a pressure that obeys the general laws of physics. It is the steady-state pressure present within the abdominal cavity.

IAP changes during respiration, increasing during inspiration and decreasing during expiration.

The basics of IAP history, abdominal anatomy and fluid physics are the main subjects of this chapter.

(Very) brief history of IAP

The timeline of IAP science is shown in Figure 1.1.

Poiseuille (1797–1869) was the first to measure pressures in confined body regions with mathematical accuracy. How we measure physiological pressures has evolved over the centuries, with much emphasis placed on arterial blood pressure.

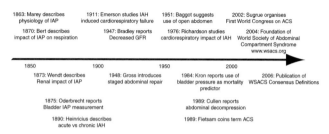

Figure 1.1

The Frenchman Etienne-Jules Marey (1830–1904) stated that 'effects' produced in the thorax by respiration are inverse to those present in the abdomen. Paul Bert (1833–1886), another Frenchman, measured pressures through tubes inserted in the trachea and rectum while working in Claude Bernard's laboratory. He described elevation of IAP during inspiration, explaining that this was caused by diaphragmatic descent.

Haven Emerson (1874–1957), a physician educated at Harvard, published his epoch-making results of IAP measurements in 1911. He developed an apparatus for direct intraperitoneal pressure measurements and found the pressure to be equal in different parts of the abdomen. Hence the abdomen was considered primarily fluid in character, following Pascal's Law. He associated cardiovascular collapse with very high IAPs and showed that drainage of ascitic fluid led to cardiac recovery.

In 1946, it was demonstrated that the magnitude of pressure at various levels in the abdomen is related to the height of the hydrostatic column of abdominal contents above the point of measurement. In other words, it was recognized that the abdomen behaved as a hydraulic system and the pressures within were hydrostatic in nature.

These findings were later challenged when it was found that IAP measured at four different sites in the abdomen were not homogeneous and that this pressure difference disappeared when the abdomen was filled with 2 litres of normal saline.

Subsequent studies concluded that there were three factors affecting IAP: gravity, uniform compression and shear deformation. Uniform compression, such as abdominal contraction, diaphragmatic contraction, mechanical ventilation, rib cage excursions and abdominal binding, result in spatially homogeneous changes in pressure that can be superimposed on the gravitational gradients.

Figure 1.2 presents the relationship between IAV, C-abd and IAP. The direction of the movement associated with the sole

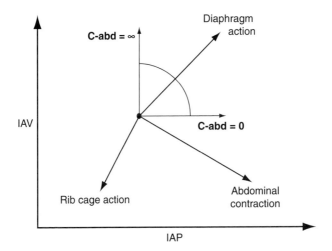

Figure 1.2

action of the rib cage inspiratory muscles, abdominal expiratory muscles and the diaphragm are shown.

The abdominal wall

The abdomen can be considered as a closed box with some parts that are rigid (spine, pelvis and costal arch) and some flexible (abdominal wall and diaphragm). The degree of flexibility of the abdominal wall (affected by multiple factors such as obesity, tissue oedema and muscle relaxants – all explained in Chapter 22) and the specific intrinsic weight of the abdominal contents (owing to solid organs such as the liver, the presence of fluid such as ascites, and the various part of the bowel) will determine the pressure at a given point.

The position of the body (prone, supine, Trendelenburg, etc.) will have an impact on IAP.

The abdominal wall forms the outer margins, extending from the thoracic cage to the pelvis. It is made of at least seven layers: the skin, subcutaneous fat, deep fascia, abdominal muscles, transverse fascia, extraperitoneal fat and the parietal peritoneum. Most of it is muscle, as shown in Figure 1.3.

Basics of fluid physics – all about pressure

Pressure is the force per unit area, and is expressed in N/m^2 in the SI system. Fluid pressure is the pressure at some point within a fluid, and can occur in an open or closed environment.

Pressure in open conditions can usually be approximated as the pressure in 'static' or non-moving conditions. The pressure

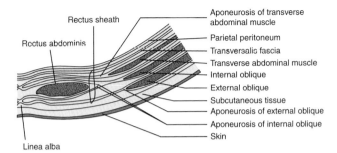

Figure 1.3

at any given point of a non-moving (static) fluid is called the
hydrostatic pressure and conforms to the principles of fluid
statics described by Blaise Pascal (1623–1662). Another name
for the unit of pressure is the Pascal (Pa): 1 Pa is $1 \, \text{N/m}^2$.

Pascal's Law, or the principle of transmission of
fluid-pressure, states: 'the pressure exerted anywhere in a
confined incompressible fluid is transmitted equally in
all directions throughout the fluid such that the pressure ratio
(initial difference) remains the same'.

This means that pressure will remain the same even if
additional pressure is applied on the fluid at some point. The
best example of this is shown in Figure 1.4, illustrating the force
exerted by a piston.

Therefore Pascal's Law can be interpreted as stating that any
change in pressure applied at any given point of the fluid is
transmitted undiminished throughout, as shown in Figure 1.4.

The difference of pressure between two points at different
heights (h1 and h2) is given by the formula shown in Figure 1.5.
The intuitive explanation of this formula is that the change in

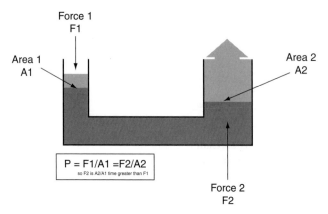

Figure 1.4

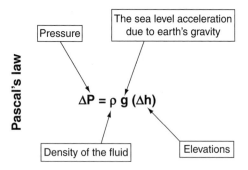

Figure 1.5

pressure between two elevations is caused by the weight of the fluid between the elevations. This means that in different body positions the hydrostatic pressure, force of gravity, is responsible for the change in pressure measured in those positions.

The IAV will exert a certain IAP on the compartment walls that will be mainly determined by C-abd. The abdominal contents are primarily fluid in character. Closed bodies of fluid are either 'static', when the fluid is not moving, or 'dynamic', when the fluid is moving. The pressure in closed conditions conforms to the principles of fluid statics by Blaise Pascal.

The abdomen at times behaves as a hydraulic system when the viscera are not subjected to shearing forces. Shearing forces are the strain in the structure of a substance, with layers laterally shifting in relation to each other, and this occurs in the abdomen. This is dependent on the shape and stability of the tissues and the degree of deformation. It is associated with spatially diverse pressure gradients. It is the relative importance of these individual factors that will ultimately determine if the abdomen behaves as a liquid-filled container.

To keep it simple, we assume that the impact of shear deformation on the measurement of IAP is probably not significant in the fully sedated mechanically ventilated patient with sepsis, capillary leak and a positive fluid balance, with or without neuromuscular blocking agents. It might not be the same in the athlete swimming through a cold swimming pool.

The relation between IAP and IAV – compliance and elastance

The relationship between pressure and volume can be expressed by the analysis of pressure–volume (P/V) curves. The same is done in respiratory physiology. The relation between IAP and IAV is the abdominal compliance (C-abd) and is calculated by the change in volume over the change in pressure (Figure 1.6).

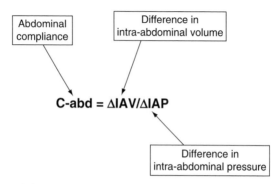

Figure 1.6

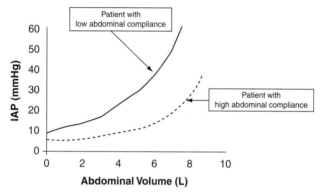

Figure 1.7

The relation between IAV and IAP is curvilinear, with an initial linear part followed by an exponential increase once a critical volume is reached, as shown in Figure 1.7.

The linear part of the abdominal pressure–volume relationship is the elastance (E-abd; Figure 1.8). In humans it was found that body weight, body mass index (BMI) and the use

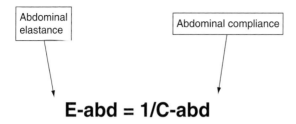

Figure 1.8

of pharmacological muscle relaxation influences the baseline pressure (called Pv_0) whereas age, pregnancy and previous abdominal surgery affects the elastance (or the slope of the initial portion of the abdominal P/V loop). This initial part of the curvilinear relationship between IAV and IAP has been studied in patients undergoing laparoscopic surgery and the elastance measured at 3 mmHg/1000 mL when Pv_0 was measured at around 5 mmHg.

It has been shown that the higher the initial IAP the greater the variation in IAP will be for the same added volume or pressure, as shown in Figure 1.9.

It has been known for a long time that effects produced in the thorax by respiration are inverse to those present in the abdomen, as shown in Figure 1.10.

The C-abd can be estimated by looking at the changes in IAP during mechanical ventilation: a low C-abd is characterized by large respiratory swings and this could help to identify patients at risk of the detrimental effects associated with elevated IAP. The observed respiratory variations are dependent on the respiratory setting and the tidal volume excursions.

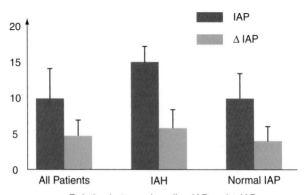

Figure 1.9

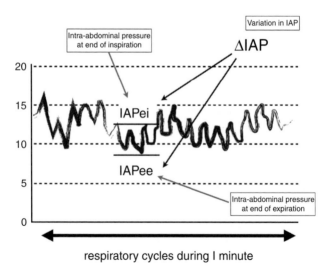

Figure 1.10

Key points

- The abdomen is a closed anatomical space.
- The abdominal contents are primarily fluid in character.
- Pascal's Law states that any change in pressure applied at any given point of the fluid is transmitted undiminished throughout the fluid. This means that IAP can be measured by way of different (in)direct routes.
- IAV will exert a certain IAP on the compartment walls that will be mainly determined by C-abd.
- The relationship between IAV and IAP is curvilinear, with an initial linear part followed by an exponential increase once a critical volume is reached.

FURTHER READING

De Keulenaer BL, De Waele JJ, Powell B, Malbrain ML. What is normal intra-abdominal pressure and how is it affected by positioning, body mass and positive end-expiratory pressure? *Intensive Care Medicine* 2009; 35(6): 969–76.

Emerson H. Intra-abdominal pressures. *Archives of Internal Medicine* 1911; 7: 754–84.

van Ramshorst GH, Salih M, Hop WC *et al.* Noninvasive assessment of intra-abdominal pressure by measurement of abdominal wall tension. *The Journal of Surgical Research* 2011; 171(1): 240–4.

Chapter 2

Definitions

Introduction

For any pathophysiological entity, a common nomenclature and definitions are essential for effective clinical communication and appraisal of the scientific literature.

Consensus definitions have been proposed for intra-abdominal hypertension (IAH) and abdominal compartment syndrome (ACS). These definitions are now widely accepted around the world.

Use of these definitions will further improve communication and future research in this area. They will need to be revised when new evidence emerges.

Background

IAH and ACS have been increasingly recognized as causes of significant morbidity and mortality over the past decade. Initially, there was little agreement regarding the definition of IAP, IAH and ACS. Comparing the results of clinical trials was difficult.

The World Society of the Abdominal Compartment Syndrome (WSACS) developed a set of consensus definitions outlining the standards for IAP measurement as well as the diagnostic criteria for IAH and ACS. These definitions are based on the best available clinical evidence and expert opinion. All good clinicians use these definitions.

Definitions

Definition 1 – IAP

IAP is the steady-state pressure concealed within the abdominal cavity.

The abdomen should be considered as a closed box with walls that may be either rigid (costal arch, spine and pelvis) or flexible (abdominal wall and diaphragm; Figure 2.1). IAP is directly affected by the volume of the solid organs or hollow viscera, the presence of ascites, blood or other space-occupying lesions (such as tumours or a gravid uterus), and the presence of conditions that limit expansion

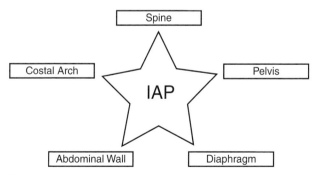

Figure 2.1

of the abdominal wall (such as burn eschars or third-space oedema).

Definition 2 – abdominal perfusion pressure (APP)

In a similar way that cerebral perfusion pressure is used for the brain, APP is a better predictor of visceral perfusion. APP can be used as an endpoint for resuscitation. APP integrates both arterial inflow (mean arterial pressure; MAP) and restrictions to venous outflow (IAP) (Figure 2.2). APP is superior to either MAP or IAP in isolation in predicting the survival of a patient suffering from IAH or ACS.

APP should be maintained above 60 mmHg to ensure adequate organ perfusion.

In patients with elevated IAP, APP is a more accurate resuscitation endpoint when compared to arterial pH, base deficit, arterial lactate or urinary output.

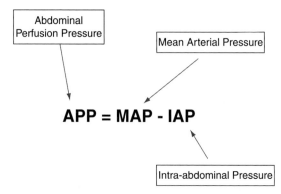

Figure 2.2

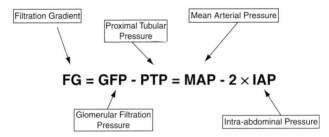

Figure 2.3

Definition 3 – filtration gradient (FG)

The FG is the mechanical force across the renal glomerulus and equals the difference between the glomerular filtration pressure (GFP) and the proximal tubular pressure (PTP) (Figure 2.3).

In the presence of IAH, PTP may be assumed to equal IAP. GFP can be estimated as MAP minus IAP.

Changes in IAP will have a greater impact than changes in MAP on renal function and urine production. This is why oliguria is one of the first signs of IAH.

Definition 4 – units of measurements and reference

IAP should be expressed in mmHg and measured at end-expiration in a strict supine position. The point of reference for the pressure measurement is the mid-axillary line, i.e. the pressure transducer must be zeroed at the level of the mid-axillary line (Figure 2.4). The upper dotted line indicates the level of the symphysis, the middle dotted line indicates the phlebostatic axis. The lowest (bold) line indicates the

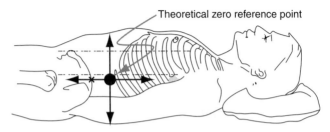

Figure 2.4

midaxillary line and the 'X' indicates the crossing with the iliac crest and this, by consensus, is the WSACs zero reference level. The operator should ascertain that abdominal muscles are not contracted. These key principles must be followed to ensure accurate and reproducible measurements.

IAP measurements are essential to the diagnosis of IAH/ACS. Physical examination is notoriously poor at identifying increased IAP.

IAP varies with respiration and is most consistently measured at end-expiration. Changes in body position (i.e. supine, prone, head of bed elevated) and the presence of both abdominal and bladder detrusor muscle contractions have been demonstrated to impact upon the accuracy of IAP measurements.

Various transducer 'zero reference' points have been suggested for IAP measurement, including the symphysis pubis, the phlebostatic axis (located at the fourth intercostal space and midway of the anterior–posterior diameter of the chest) or the mid-axillary line. Each of these results in different IAP values within the same patient.

Early studies using water manometers reported results in cmH_2O while subsequent studies using electronic pressure transducers reported IAP in mmHg (conversion is $1\ mmHg = 1.36\ cmH_2O$).

Definition 5 – reference standard

The reference standard for intermittent IAP measurement is through the bladder with a maximal instillation volume of 25 mL of sterile saline.

Multiple studies have demonstrated that instillation of volumes in excess of 25 mL will artificially increase IAP when using the bladder technique (described in Chapter 3). This leads to erroneous measurements and inappropriate treatment. Some studies have suggested that volumes as low as 2 mL are sufficient.

Definition 6 – normal IAP

Normal IAP is approximately 5–7 mmHg in critically ill adults

IAP can be subatmospheric or equal to 0 mmHg.

Morbid obesity or pregnancy may be associated with asymptomatic IAP elevations of up to 15 mmHg. These are generally well tolerated owing to their chronicity and slow onset. The same pressure occurring acutely will impact significantly on organ perfusion. Recent abdominal surgery, sepsis, organ failure and the need for mechanical ventilation are associated with elevated IAP.

The clinical importance of any change in IAP must always be assessed in view of the baseline IAP for the individual patient.

Definition 7 – IAH

IAH is defined by a sustained or repeated pathological elevation of IAP $\geq$ 12 mmHg.

This value has been the subject of many debates. Pathological IAP is a continuum ranging from mild, asymptomatic elevations in IAP to marked elevations that have grave consequences on virtually every organ system in the body.

The majority of studies show that visceral organ perfusion starts to decrease when IAP is at around 10–15 mmHg. It is at this level that cardiac, renal, hepatic and gastrointestinal perfusion becomes compromised and anaerobic metabolism kicks in. This is rapidly followed by organ dysfunction and failure.

Definition 8 – IAH grades

Patients with prolonged untreated elevations in IAP manifest inadequate perfusion and subsequent organ failure. The more severe the degree of IAH, the more urgent is the need to reduce the damaging pressure (either medically or surgically). Grading systems help to improve communication and standardize clinical research (Table 2.1).

Table 2.1 Grades of IAH

Grade	Range of IAP (mmHg)
1	12–15 mmHg
2	16–20 mmHg
3	21–25 mmHg
4	> 25 mmHg

Definition 9 – ACS

ACS is defined as a sustained IAP > 20 mmHg (with or without an APP < 60 mmHg) that is associated with new organ dysfunction and/or failure.

ACS is best remembered as the presence of significant IAH with organ failure. Failure to recognize and appropriately treat ACS is uniformly fatal whereas prevention and timely intervention are associated with marked improvement in organ function and patient survival.

In contrast to IAH, ACS is not graded, but rather considered an 'all or nothing' phenomenon. There are three different types of ICH/ACS, and these constitute definitions 10, 11 and 12 of the consensus.

Definition 10 – primary ACS

Primary ICH/ACS is a condition associated with injury or disease in the abdominal and pelvic regions that requires early surgical or invasive radiological intervention.

Primary ICH/ACS is characterized by an acute or subacute IAH of relatively brief duration occurring as a result of pathologies listed in Table 2.2.

Primary ICH/ACS is most commonly seen in the traumatically injured or postoperative surgical patient.

Definition 11 – secondary ACS

Secondary ICH/ACS refers to conditions that do not originate from the abdominopelvic region.

Table 2.2 Possible causes of primary ICH/ACS

Abdominal trauma

Ruptured abdominal aortic aneurysm

Haemoperitoneum

Acute pancreatitis

Secondary peritonitis

Retroperitoneal haemorrhage

Liver transplantation

Table 2.3 Possible causes of secondary ICH/ACS

Sepsis

Capillary leak

Major burns

Massive fluid resuscitation

Secondary ICH/ACS is characterized by subacute or chronic IAH that develops owing to extra-abdominal pathology such as those listed in Table 2.3.

Secondary ICH/ACS is most commonly seen in the medical or burn patient.

Definition 12 – recurrent ACS

Recurrent ACS refers to the condition in which ACS redevelops following previous surgical or medical treatment of primary or secondary ACS.

Recurrent ACS is when the ACS symptoms occur again after resolution of an earlier episode of either primary or secondary

ACS. It occurs during recovery from IAH and/or ACS and represents a 'second-hit' phenomenon.

Recurrent ACS can occur despite an open abdomen. It can be a new ACS episode following closure of the abdominal cavity.

Recurrent ACS is associated with high morbidity and mortality.

The future of the definitions

The current WSACS definitions are constantly being reviewed and re-evaluated and might be revised as needed to improve their clinical usefulness and accuracy.

Key points

- IAP is an important physiological measurement.
- Consensus definitions must be used.
- Both IAP and APP should be monitored during patient resuscitation.
- IAH = IAP ≥ 12 mmHg.
- ACS = IAP > 20 mmHg with organ failure.

FURTHER READING

Cheatham ML, Malbrain MLNG, Kirkpatrick A *et al*. Results from the conference of experts on intra-abdominal hypertension and abdominal compartment syndrome. Part II: Recommendations. *Intensive Care Medicine* 2007; 33: 951–62.

Malbrain MLNG, Cheatham ML, Kirkpatrick A *et al.* Results from the conference of experts on intra-abdominal hypertension and abdominal compartment syndrome. Part I: Definitions. *Intensive Care Medicine* 2006; 32: 1722–32.

Chapter 3

Principles of IAP management

Measure IAP at the end of expiration

IAP should be measured at end-expiration (IAPee), with the patient supine and ensuring that there is no abdominal muscle activity.

This is important in spontaneously breathing patients as it affects the normal pressure–volume curve. Forceful expiration will overestimate IAP.

Figure 3.1 illustrates a trace recorded during relaxed spontaneous breathing (panel A) and during forced expiration with abdominal muscle contraction (panel B).

Confirmation of correct IAP measurement can be done by inspection of the variations observed during ventilation. Gently applied oscillations to the abdomen should be transmitted and seen on the monitor with a quick return to baseline, as illustrated in Figure 3.2.

IAP is (usually) measured in the bladder

The bladder is in the abdominal compartment. The intravesical pressure is equal to the IAP as the pressure is uniform in the abdomen. Measurement of IAP in the bladder (intravesical) has

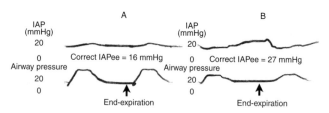

Figure 3.1

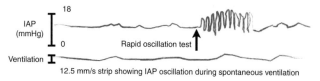

Figure 3.2

emerged as a reliable method and the gold standard for indirect measurement.

IAP may be falsely elevated in the case of an extrinsic compression of the bladder such as is observed in patients with pelvic haematoma or other space-occupying lesion in the pelvis.

As long as there is not a high volume of liquid in the bladder, the detrusor muscle does not generate any tension and therefore does not influence IAP measurements. The bladder compliance may be affected when normal volumes are small, such as in anuric patients with chronic renal failure. A falsely high IAP can be read because the detrusor contracts when stretched by even a small volume of injectate. This phenomenon can be observed in patients who have had prolonged bladder catheter drainage. In these conditions, intragastric IAP measurement may be preferable.

IAP can be measured through routes other than the bladder

The IAP is uniform throughout the abdomen and it can therefore be measured at any intra-abdominal location. The limitations to other routes are practical.

The stomach is the second most conveniently accessible site.

Alternatives could include the rectum and uterus, both accessible with a tube.

A measure can also be obtained from the inside of the inferior vena cava using an intravenous catheter.

Any catheter located in the abdomen, such as postoperative drains or peritoneal dialysis catheters, can be used for IAP measurement.

IAP can be measured with fluid-filled or air-filled systems

Fluid-filled systems use fluids to conduct the pressure to the transducer, and air-filled systems use air. Both systems can be used for IAP measurement.

Air-filled systems are based on an air-filled balloon positioned in the abdominal cavity, e.g. in the stomach. When using air-filled systems, it is not necessary to have the transducer at the mid-axillary level, but regular zeroing of the pressure transducer is still required.

IAP should be measured against a reference level

In theory, the correct reference level to use is the mid-bladder level, i.e. the level of the tip of the urinary catheter. In practice, this level cannot be identified at the bedside.

Previously, the pubic symphysis was recommended as a reference line. It proved that the exact localization of the pubic symphysis was different when assessed by different physicians, owing to differences in patient body morphology. This led to variation in IAP.

To avoid problems of localization, the mid-axillary line was suggested as the reference line. The mid-axillary line anatomically projects at the level of the mid-bladder in most patients, and is easier to identify in critically ill patients.

To monitor IAP reliably and compare successive values, it is advisable to put a mark on the patient's skin at the moment of the first IAP measurement, so all agree where the mid-axillary line is.

Figure 3.3 illustrates the anatomical location of the different zero reference points in relation to the theoretical zero reference, i.e. the mid-abdominal position. The location of different zero reference positions (suprapubic, iliac crest and phlebostatic axis) and their relative position to the theoretical zero reference are shown in a patient with normal shape and normal IAP. Figure 3.4 shows the same in a patient with a distended abdomen and increased IAP. In this case, the phlebostatic axis is closest to the theoretical zero reference in the supine position.

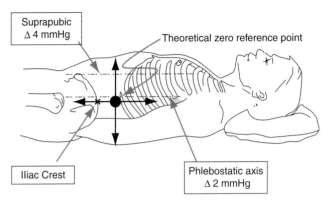

Figure 3.3

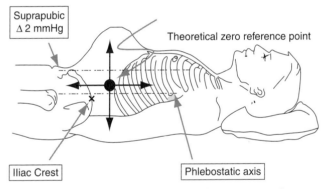

Figure 3.4 X represents midaxillary line where it crosses the iliac crest.

Instillation of fluid in the bladder is required

In the enthusiasm of the early days of IAP measurement, clinicians used high instillation volumes (sometimes as much as 250 mL). It is now known that volumes above 25 mL may increase the IAP reading because of increased tension of the detrusor muscle.

A small volume (10–20 mL) has proven reliable to measure IAP.

In adults, the recommended instillation volume is 25 mL maximum. It is 1 mL/kg, up to a maximum of 20 mL, in children.

The temperature of the instillation fluid should be controlled

If the temperature of the instillation fluid is lower than the body temperature, the detrusor muscle may contract, resulting in the recording of an erroneously high IAP.

It is thought that this effect is negligible if small instillation volumes are used.

The patient's body position is important

Supine versus semi-recumbent position

The IAP is 3–5 mmHg higher when measured in the semi-recumbent position (head of the bed elevated at 30°). It will be 6–9 mmHg higher if the bed is elevated at 45°. This effect is greater in patients with high BMI.

This is explained by the descent of intra-abdominal contents when the head of the bed is elevated, and the additional pressure this exerts on the bladder. Positioning will have a profound effect on IAP if the patient has a poorly compliant abdomen.

It is therefore best to measure IAP in the supine position throughout the day.

To accommodate the conflicting demands of IAP optimal measurement and best nursing practice (patients in the semi-recumbent position to avoid aspiration), the head of the bed should not be elevated to more than 30° when patients present with IAH.

Prone position

Prone positioning will either exacerbate or improve IAH, depending on the technique used. It is therefore important to describe what was done when reporting such patients. Supporting the pelvis and rib cage to unload the abdomen should be considered in patients with IAH and high BMI, as compression of the abdomen will increase IAP.

Other positions

Figure 3.5 illustrates how different positions will affect the reading of IAP when measured via the bladder. The observed effects will be dependent on body shape, baseline IAP and the compliance of the abdominal wall.

It is still under discussion whether the variation in IAP caused by position is always a true increase in IAP or simply a measurement error.

The effect of positive end expiratory pressure (PEEP) on IAP

Increasing the PEEP may decrease the compliance of the diaphragm and lead to changes in IAP.

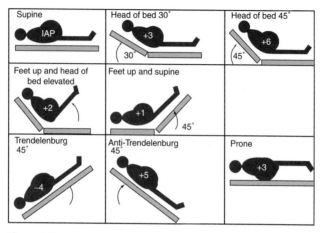

Figure 3.5

Increasing PEEP to 15 cmH$_2$O in patients with a baseline IAP below 12 mmHg results in a mild increase of about 1–2 mmHg. The effect of an increase in PEEP will be greater if the baseline IAP is 12 mmHg or above, owing to the decreased compliance of the abdominal wall. However, these effects are not consistent and some studies have shown less effects of PEEP on IAP in patients with IAH.

Key points

- IAP should be measured at end-expiration, with the patient in the supine position and ensuring that there is no abdominal muscle activity.
- Intravesicular IAP measurement is convenient and the most widely used technique.

- Where the mid-axillary line crosses the iliac crest is the recommended reference level for transvesicular IAP measurement; marking this level on the patient increases reproducibility.
- Instillation volume and temperature may affect IAP readings.
- When the head of the bed is elevated to 30°, IAP is increased.
- PEEP only minimally affects IAP.
- Protocols for IAP measurement should be developed for each ICU based on the local available tools and equipment.

FURTHER READING

De Keulenaer BL, De Waele JJ, Powell B, Malbrain ML. What is normal intra-abdominal pressure and how is it affected by positioning, body mass and positive end-expiratory pressure? *Intensive Care Medicine* 2009; 35: 969–76.

De Waele JJ, De laet I, Malbrain ML. Rational intra-abdominal pressure monitoring: how to do it? *Acta Clinica Belgica* (Suppl.) 2007; 62(1): 16–25.

Verzilli D, Constantin JM, Sebbane M *et al.* Positive end-expiratory pressure affects the value of intra-abdominal pressure in acute lung injury/acute respiratory distress syndrome patients: a pilot study. *Critical Care* 2010; 14(4): R137.

Chapter 4

Systems available to measure IAP

Introduction

IAP measurement has evolved considerably over the years. Home-made systems set up by the handy clinician were the only option before the advent of reliable and reproducible methods.

The need for self-assembly has been a considerable obstacle to the widespread implementation of IAP measurement in clinical practice.

Systems to measure IAP are now simpler, and some allow continuous IAP measurement.

Clinical estimation of IAP

Clinical examination of the abdomen is definitely not sensitive enough, and is proven not to detect IAH.

Extreme cases of ACS can probably be diagnosed clinically, but the effect of therapeutic interventions can only be monitored with adequate IAP monitoring.

The abdominal perimeter is not a surrogate of IAP and cannot be used to detect patients at risk for IAH and ACS, or monitor any treatment effect.

Measurement of IAP is safe

Many methods to measure IAP are safe as long as an appropriate technique is used.

Concerns have been expressed about the risk of urinary tract infection when injecting urine back from the catheter to the bladder, but no studies have been able to detect a negative effect.

Concerns exist about the patient's position. While short periods in the supine position are usually well tolerated, it is accepted that IAP can be monitored when the patient is kept in a 30° head-up position (the IAP measured tends to be 3–5 mmHg higher in that position, as discussed in Chapter 3).

Measurement of IAP is reproducible

IAP has to be measured in the correct position using a reliable technique. Appropriate care should be taken to use the same reference level in all measurements when using fluid-filled systems. For practical purposes and to ensure accurate monitoring, this level should be marked on the patient's skin when the first measurement is made.

Routes for IAP measurements

IAP measurement can be direct or indirect. Direct measurement is used when the catheter or balloon is located directly in the peritoneal cavity. Direct measurement is only rarely performed. Patients with a catheter for peritoneal dialysis have such a measurement performed easily. Surgeons can insert balloon catheters intraoperatively, such as during laparoscopic surgery (during which IAP should not exceed 15 mmHg). Indirect measurement is when the catheter or balloon is inserted in a cavity within the abdominal wall.

The division between direct and indirect is somewhat artificial as the pressure is equal in all points of the abdominal cavity (explained in Chapter 1). An indirect measurement of IAP is a true estimate. In practice, we do not differentiate direct from indirect.

Transvesicular route

The bladder is readily accessible in most patients at risk for IAH and ACS and the transvesicular or bladder route is frequently used.

The bladder is considered to have a compliant wall without any tension when it is drained or filled with minimal volumes. The intravesicular pressure (IVP) is an adequate and reliable estimation of IAP.

The height of the urine column in the urine drainage tubing will affect this measure, hence the need for a good technique. This means injecting a known amount of fluid to the drained bladder.

The bladder detrusor muscle can contract when stretched by a large amount of fluid, with a subsequent increase in IVP and an overestimation of IAP. These contractions only last for up to 30 seconds. Cold can trigger these contractions. It is therefore ideal to use a small amount of liquid (<25 mL) at body temperature.

Transgastric route

The stomach is easy to access and is usually located in the abdomen.

The high volume of the stomach and its large openings at both ends preclude the instillation of fluid. In patients tolerating enteral nutrition, IAP could theoretically be measured via the nasogastric tube. In other patients, a continuous flow is needed to allow IAP measurement.

Balloon catheters are used in the stomach and allow continuous measurement. Recent data show that intragastric pressure (IGP) can be assessed by measuring the height of the enteral nutrition column in the nasogastric tube.

Alternative routes

IAP has been measured using rectal or uterine catheters. These are not always practical for continued IAP measurement in critically ill patients.

The inferior vena cava pressure is an alternative route in patients with femoral venous catheters. This method seems valid when the values of IAP are above 15–20 mmHg, but it is unknown if it is reliable at normal IAP.

Modalities of IAP measurements

IAP measurement is done intermittently or continuously.

Continuous IAP measurement has multiple advantages, listed in Table 4.1. In some cases, IAP values can be

Table 4.1 Benefits of continuous IAP measurement

Reduction in workload at the bedside

Real-time measurement

Contemporaneous review of interventions aimed at decreasing IAP

Possibility to alert immediately when IAP increases

continuously viewed on the bedside monitoring screen, if allowed by the manufacturer.

Available methods for IAP measurement

Intermittent IAP measurement

Transvesicular: FoleyManometer™ or Uno-Meter Abdo-Pressure™

This device consists of a tube connected between the patient's bladder catheter and the urine collector. The FoleyManometer™ or Uno-Meter Abdo-Pressure™ tube is then elevated, allowing the urine to return to the bladder. The resulting column of fluid is the IAP (Figure 4.1).

This device allows the pressure to equilibrate with the atmospheric pressure in the lumen above the urine column when the clamp below a biofilter is released. The IAP can be read directly from the tubing in mmHg after a maximal amount of 10 mL of fresh urine is returned to the bladder.

Details about the FoleyManometer™ can be found on http://www.holtech-medical.com.

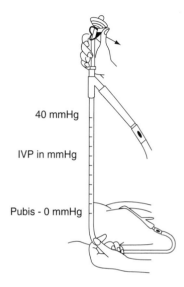

40 mmHg

IVP in mmHg

Pubis - 0 mmHg

With permission, Holtech Medical

Figure 4.1

Details about the Uno-Meter Abdo-Pressure™ can be found on http://iap.unomedical-urology.com.

Transvesicular: Harahill method

The Harahill method is based on the same principle as the FoleyManometer™, but uses the available tubing connected to the urine collector.

This technique can only be applied if a pressure release valve is available on the urine collector; if not, the pressure above the urine column may be negative, not allowing the urine to drop and leading to an overestimation of IAP (see Figure 4.2).

This is an important obstacle to the use of this method, as most collectors do not have this pressure release valve. In these cases, the tubing must be disconnected to allow the urine to descend and equilibrate with the pressure.

The urine column should be measured using a measuring tape in centimetres, and converted to mmHg (dividing the

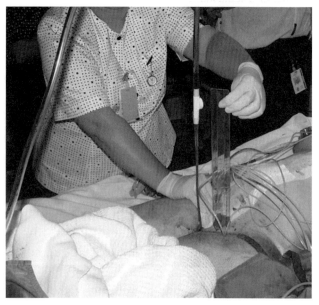

Figure 4.2

height in centimetres by 1.36, assuming that urine has the same density as water).

Transvesicular: AbViser™ IAP Monitoring Kit

The AbViser™ series of IAP monitoring kits consist of an interface that is interposed between the urinary catheter and the urine collection system. During IAP measurement, turning the valve allows fluid to be instilled into the bladder, creating a fluid column from the bladder to a pressure transducer. The AbViser™ AutoValve™ has an automatic valve that allows IAP measurement with minimal additional manipulations (see Figure 4.3).

A special adaptor is separately available which allows IAP measurement in neonates and small children.

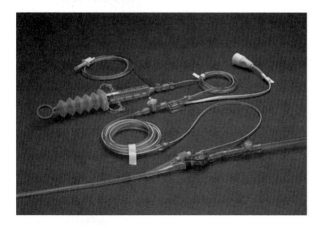

With permission, Abviser

Figure 4.3

Details about the AbViser™ series can be found at http://www.convatec.com/products.

Transvesicular: Bard IAP® Monitoring Device

The Bard IAP® monitoring device consists of an interface interposed between the urinary catheter and the urinary collection system. During IAP measurement, turning the valve clamps the urinary drainage tube and allows fluid to be instilled into the bladder, creating a fluid column from the bladder to a pressure transducer.

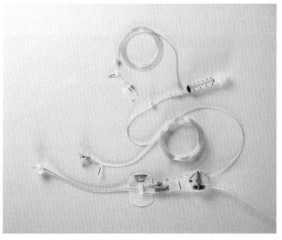

With permission, CR Bard

Figure 4.4

Details about the Bard IAP® monitoring device can be found at http://www.bardmedical.com/products.

Transvesicular: Biometrix

Urimetrix™, Biometrix's comprehensive product line for urine drainage management, includes high level urine meters, Foley catheters with temperature sensor and IAP sets with accurate pressure transducer monitoring. Urimetrix™ is easy to use, with efficient emptying time and needle-free sampling port. More details can be found at http://www.biometrixmedical.com/Products/56/Urimetrix™.

Transvesicular: PreOx IAP Adapter

The PreOx IAP adapter consists of an interface which is interposed between the Foley catheter and the urinary collection system. It consists of a barbed adapter with integrated funnel connector and pressure measuring line for easy setup between bladder catheter and urine bag (see Figure 4.5). A sliding clamp premounted at a defined position allows reproducible and comparable values for each pressure measurement. During IAP measurement, turning the valve clamps the urinary drainage tube and allows fluid to be instilled into the bladder, creating a fluid column from the bladder to a pressure transducer.

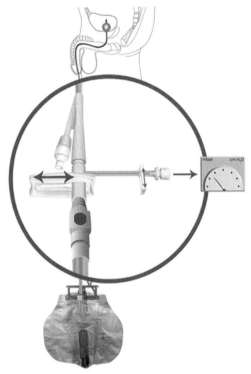

With permission, PreOx

Figure 4.5

Details about the PreOx IAP adapter device can be found at http://www.preox.de.

Transgastric: gastric tube or Collee method

This method uses a nasogastric or gastrostomy tube, and is comparable to most of the transvesicular methods.

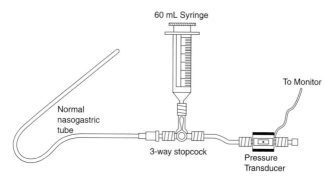

Figure 4.6

A pressure transducer is connected to the lumen of the nasogastric tube, and, after instillation of 100–200 mL of saline into the stomach and zeroing the pressure transducer, the IAP can be read from the monitor. The stomach should be completely empty (including air) before this method is used.

Transgastric: gastric balloon method

An oesophageal balloon catheter is inserted into the oesophagus and connected to a pressure transducer. Using a syringe, 1 mL of air is introduced into the balloon and, after zeroing to atmospheric pressure, the IAP can be read from the monitor. The position of the balloon can be checked using an oscillation test or by observing the pressure readings from the catheter.

The air from the balloon is reabsorbed after a few hours so recalibration is necessary. This is illustrated in the lower panel of Figure 4.7. The reabsorption of air is recorded as a loss of IAP signal.

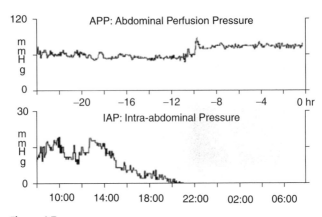

Figure 4.7

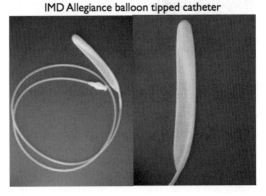

IMD Allegiance balloon tipped catheter

Figure 4.8

Figure 4.8 shows an IMD Allegiance balloon-tipped catheter; Figure 4.9 the Ackrad balloon-tipped catheter; Figure 4.10 the Datex tonometer catheter; and Figure 4.11 the NutriVent™ catheter with two balloons.

Ackrad balloon tipped catheter

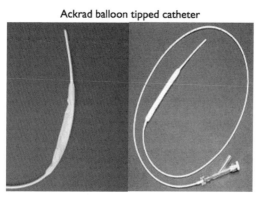

Figure 4.9

Datex tonometer catheter

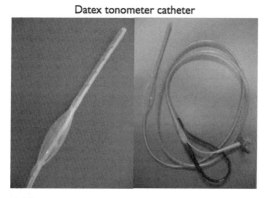

Figure 4.10

Continuous IAP measurement

Continuous transvesicular IAP measurement

IAP can be measured continuously using a 3-way Foley
catheter, with one lumen connected to a pressure transducer

Nutrivent catheter with 2 balloons

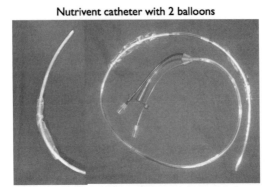

Figure 4.11

Continuous trans-vesicular IAP measurement

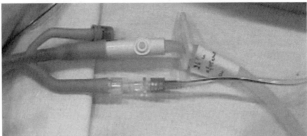

Figure 4.12

(see Figure 4.12). A continuous flow of saline (e.g. from an infusion pump) is required at a low speed (2–4 mL/h) in the dedicated lumen for reliable IAP measurement.

The issue of draining urine and measuring IAP at the same time needs to be solved; this is analogous to the brain where one cannot measure the intracranial pressure (ICP) and drain the cerebrospinal fluid at the same time.

Once a urine column is formed from the bladder to the collection bag, a negative suction force can be created, causing underestimation of the real IAP. Air bubbles on the other hand can cause an overestimation of the real IAP.

Continuous IAP monitoring – CiMON (Pulsion Medical Systems)

CiMON provides continuous IAP monitoring via a special nasogastric probe combining feeding, decompression and IAP measurement function (Figure 4.13). The IAP is measured via a small air-filled balloon located at the distal tip of the CiMON probe.

The catheter is connected to a specific monitor that allows continuous IAP and APP measurements and monitoring. In the future, new probes are likely to be available in the form of nasojejunal 3-lumen postpyloric feeding tubes or even 4-lumen probes equipped with an oesophageal and gastric balloon for transdiaphragmatic pressure measurement.

Details about the CiMON device can be found at http://www.pulsion.com.

The IAP-Catheter and IAP-Monitor (Spiegelberg)

The IAP-Catheter is introduced like a nasogastric tube. It is equipped with an air-pouch at the tip. The catheter has one

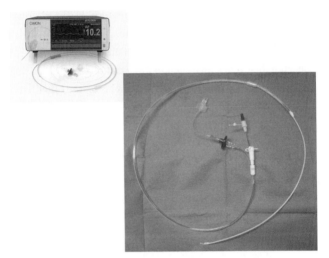

Figure 4.13

lumen that connects the air-pouch with an IAP-Monitor and one lumen that takes the guidewire.

Details about the IAP-Catheter can be found at http://www. spiegelberg.de/products.

Key points

- IAP measurement techniques are safe, reproducible and accurate.
- IAP measurement techniques have greatly improved over the years, with multiple assembled kits commercially available.

• Continuous IAP measurement is simple and offers added
  values in specific situations.

FURTHER READING

Balogh Z, De Waele JJ, Malbrain ML. Continuous
    intra-abdominal pressure monitoring. *Acta Clinica Belgica
    Supplement* 2007; 62(1): 26–32.
De Waele JJ, De Laet I, Malbrain ML. Rational
    intraabdominal pressure monitoring: how to do it? *Acta
    Clinica Belgica* 2007; 62(1): 16–25.

Chapter 5

Pitfalls of IAP monitoring

Introduction

Accurate and reproducible IAP measurement is essential in the management of patients with IAH and ACS. IAH is defined as an IAP between 12 and 20 mmHg. It is therefore important to identify an accurate value to define a potential problem.

Trends in IAP may be more important in certain conditions and therefore repeated reliable IAP measurements are essential.

Clinicians involved in the care of the patient with IAH should be aware of pitfalls in the measurement of IAP. Most can easily be avoided if guidelines and protocols are properly set.

The pitfalls

Pitfalls in IAP measurement can be related to the patient, the measurement technique or the interpretation of the value obtained.

Pitfalls related to the patient

Positioning of the patient

The patient should be put in the supine position for IAP measurement. Measuring IAP with the head of the bed elevated leads to higher values, and measurements in one position should not be compared with the values obtained in another.

In some patients, it may be contraindicated to change the body position and it is accepted that IAP can be measured with the head of the bed elevated as long as the classical thresholds for IAH and ACS are not applied.

The awake patient

In awake patients, spontaneous breathing and abdominal muscle contractions (notably after abdominal surgical procedures) can influence the IAP value. This can lead to falsely elevated values in case of forced expiration or increased abdominal muscle tension.

Deep inspiration changes the classical IAP curve observed in mechanically ventilated patients, and may confuse the observer and the monitor software.

Intra-abdominal space-occupying lesions

The presence of mass in the abdomen or pelvis (e.g. haematomas in patients with pelvic fractures or spontaneous haemorrhages in the rectus sheath or muscles) may compress the bladder and lead to falsely elevated IAP values.

Obesity

Patients with BMI higher than normal have elevated IAP. Other thresholds for IAH and ACS may be applicable.

Children

Small children tend to have lower blood pressure values. IAP values will also be lower. Other thresholds for IAH and ACS may be applicable.

Pitfalls related to the measurement technique

Zero reference level

Most of the techniques to monitor IAP use fluid-filled systems for pressure transduction. Correct calibration of the transducer is of paramount importance for reliable IAP measurement. It is important to use the correct zero reference level, as described in Chapter 2. It is advisable to mark this level on the patient, and the transducer should be zeroed before each IAP measurement.

Gastric route

When measuring IAP by the oesogastric route, it is important to consider rhythmic changes caused by peristaltic waves. Gastric dilatation can also affect readings.

Intrathoracic positioning of the balloon can be excluded from the analysis of the waveform: the pressure elevation during inspiration is mostly dampened when correctly positioned; and the oscillation test – which consists of gently tapping on the abdomen and should result in an oscillating curve on the monitor – may be helpful. Gastric pressure IAP tracings often include cardiac rhythm artefacts.

Infusion volume

Injection in the bladder of volumes larger than 25 mL leads to overestimation of IAP. Although these differences are usually small, they can be clinically significant. These appear to be more relevant after several days of urinary bladder drainage and in patients with reduced abdominal wall compliance.

Infusion temperature

Cold fluids may cause the bladder detrusor muscle to contract and lead to elevated intravesicular pressure measurements.

Frequency of IAP measurement

IAP may rapidly change in critically ill patients, most importantly in patients with intra-abdominal pathology. When IAP is only measured once or twice a day, these changes will be unnoticed or only diagnosed at a late stage. IAP measurement every 4 hours, or more frequently in unstable patients, is recommended. Single measurements of IAP during critical illness in patients at risk should be discouraged. Instillation of saline in the bladder has not been associated with increased incidence of urinary tract infection. This should not be used as an argument to refrain from or stop IAP measurement.

Pitfall specific to the kit used

When using kits such as the AbViser kit with the AutoValve (Wolfe Tory Medical, USA), the valve closes after 60–120 seconds.

When using the FoleyManometer (Holtech Medical, Denmark), the amount of fluid in the tubing must be adequate. This might not be the case in oliguric patients. Insufficient volume will lead to underestimation of the IAP. This can easily be resolved by injecting 20 mL of saline in the FoleyManometer tubing.

Pitfalls related to the interpretation of data

These can be avoided by reading the whole book!

Key points

- Pitfalls in IAP measurement are multiple, and thorough knowledge of the technique used for IAP measurement is essential.
- Infusion volume for intravesicular pressure measurement should be limited to 25 mL.
- Determination of the correct zero reference level is important and should be done at the start of IAP measurement.
- Absence of abdominal muscle activity should be checked, particularly in awake patients.

FURTHER READING

Malbrain ML. Different techniques to measure intra-abdominal pressure (IAP): time for a critical re-appraisal. *Intensive Care Medicine* 2004; 30(3): 357–71.

**Underlying predisposing conditions:
when to worry?**

Chapter 6

Decreased abdominal compliance

What is abdominal compliance?

In analogy to the respiratory system, any change in intra-abdominal volume (IAV) is accompanied by a change in intra-abdominal pressure (IAP). The relationship between both is defined as abdominal wall compliance (C-abd) and this has been described in Chapter 1.

Increased IAP is caused by an increase in IAV, a decrease in C-abd or a combination of both. Changes in C-abd are usually because of changes in the anterolateral abdominal wall and, to a lesser extent, because of changes in intrathoracic pressure (diaphragm and rib cage).

C-abd is calculated by the change in volume over the change in pressure ($\Delta V/\Delta P$). It cannot be readily measured or calculated at the bedside and its exact value is of limited importance.

The abdominal pressure–volume curve has two parts: a part in which relatively large changes in volume produce only small changes in pressure (or a 'compensated' part) and a part, at higher volumes and pressures, in which small volume changes lead to large pressure changes. This part of the curve is initially linear with an increasing slope at higher pressures.

The inclination of the curve depends on C-abd. C-abd is highest at low IAP and decreases with increasing IAP.

C-abd is the derivative of the abdominal P/V curve.

Various causes of decreased C-abd have been described, but third space oedema in the abdominal wall is probably most frequently encountered.

In conditions associated with intrinsic decreased C-abd, such as scars or oedema, the abdominal P/V curve is shifted to the upper left, as shown in Figure 1.7.

Why is abdominal compliance important?

A compartment syndrome exists when the pressure in a confined anatomical space is increased and the organs or anatomical structures within the compartment are affected by the pressure increase. Usually, this happens when the volume within the compartment is increased and the walls of the compartment are rigid and unable to accommodate the extra volume. This concept can be appreciated in the skull, where relatively small amounts of cerebral oedema (or volume increase) can lead to a compartment syndrome (cerebral herniation and brain death) because the bony skull has completely rigid walls and there are few compensation mechanisms.

In the abdominal cavity, the walls of the compartment are formed by the rib cage (or the thoracic wall), the diaphragm, the pelvis, the spine with its adjacent musculature and the anterolateral abdominal wall. Among these anatomical entities, the anterolateral abdominal wall, the diaphragm and, to a certain extent, the rib cage are the most malleable or 'compliant'. The diaphragm and the rib cage cannot be viewed separately from their function in the thoracic compartment. The abdominal and thoracic compartments are closely interlinked and pressures applied to one compartment are transmitted to the other compartment. Since the diaphragm and the thoracic wall compliance are so closely related to ventilation, and these compliances are not very amenable to therapeutic intervention, the compliance of the anterolateral abdominal wall is the main interest.

Implications for clinical practice

How does decreased abdominal wall compliance lead to IAH?

The relationship between IAV and IAP behaves in a similar way to the relationship between intracerebral volume and intracranial pressure (ICP). The ICP remains constant over a relatively wide range of intracranial volumes. An increase in intracranial volume caused by cerebral oedema, haematoma or a mass will be compensated by the evacuation of cerebrospinal fluid through the foramen magnum at the base of the skull. When this compensation mechanism is exhausted, any small increase in volume produces a marked increase in ICP.

   In the abdomen fluids cannot be moved easily into another anatomical space. The abdominal wall is less rigid than the bony skull and can stretch. This keeps the IAP constant when IAV increases. When the compliance of the abdominal wall is decreased, this compensation is impaired and an increase in IAV leads to an increase in IAP.

Is this clinically important?

Some specific conditions are associated with decreased C-abd; these include abdominal eschars in burn patients, tension after abdominal wall reconstruction or restrictive abdominal bandages (see Table 6.1).

Most of the time, C-abd is decreased by oedema of the abdominal wall after massive fluid resuscitation. Large amounts of crystalloid fluid resuscitation will lead to extravasation of fluids

Table 6.1 Risk factors for the development of IAH and ACS

In the context of decreased C-abd
Mechanical ventilation, especially fighting with the ventilator and the use of accessory muscles
Use of positive end expiratory pressure (PEEP) or the presence of auto-PEEP
Basal pneumonia
High body mass index (BMI)
During pneumoperitoneum
Abdominal (vascular) surgery, especially with tight abdominal closures
Pneumatic anti-shock garments
Prone and other body positioning
Abdominal wall bleeding or rectus sheath haematomas
Correction of large hernias, gastroschisis or omphalocele
Burns with abdominal eschars
Abdominal scars
Use of abdominal velcro belt
Abdominal wall oedema after massive fluid loading during capillary leak

into the interstitial space, oedema of the bowel and of the abdominal wall. In many cases there is accumulation of free fluids in the peritoneal space. C-abd is already decreased owing to the increased IAV and will be further compromised by oedema of the abdominal wall. This is a frequent cause of secondary IAH and associated mortality.

Can I and should I measure abdominal compliance in my patient?

To calculate the exact value for C-abd one would have to add or extract a known volume to the abdomen (ΔV) and measure the resulting change in IAP (ΔP). Knowing the exact value of abdominal compliance does not provide any additional useful information. C-abd is never routinely measured or calculated in clinical practice.

It is important to grasp the C-abd concept to understand and recognize the contribution of the abdominal wall to IAH and to consider possible treatment options that influence C-abd.

In theory, C-abd could be measured at the bedside in a mechanically ventilated patient by examining the effect of gradually increasing tidal volume on IAP.

How do I know when abdominal wall compliance is decreased?

C-abd is not measured routinely in clinical practice but there are circumstances and signs pointing to decreased C-abd that can be checked at the bedside.

Decreased C-abd should be suspected in all patients receiving large amounts of resuscitation fluids, such as patients with burns, severe acute pancreatitis, septic shock, severe trauma and massive transfusion.

The presence of solutions to assist primary abdominal closure after laparotomy or material often used to prevent incisional hernias may indicate that IAP is increased in postoperative patients (Figures 6.1–6.3).

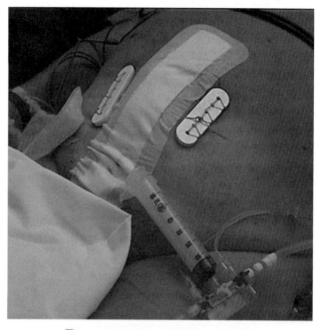

Retention sutures

Figure 6.1

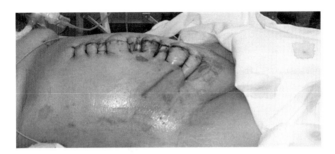

Tight abdominal closure of midline laparotomy

Figure 6.2

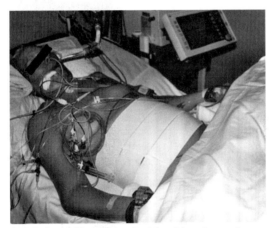

A velcro belt used to prevent incisional hernia may increase IAP

Figure 6.3

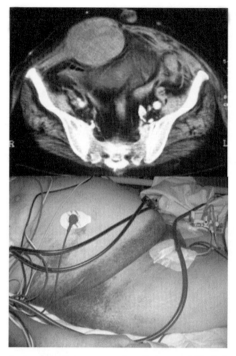

Large haematoma causing decreased C-abd

Figure 6.4

Mass lesions that directly affect the abdominal wall, such as haematomas, can affect compliance (Figure 6.4).

When IAP is measured using a pressure transducer and a pressure curve is registered, it is possible to record abdominal pressures respectively at the end of inspiration

(IAPei) and the end of expiration (IAPee). During inspiration, the diaphragm and upper abdominal organs are displaced caudally, decreasing the craniocaudal length of the abdomen. This is almost fully compensated in normal circumstances by the anterior displacement of the muscular abdominal wall. In patients with decreased C-abd, this compensation is impaired, meaning that IAP will increase markedly during inspiration. The difference between IAPei and IAPee (or ΔIAP) provides an indirect measure of abdominal wall compliance. A low ΔIAP indicates a compliant abdominal wall and a high ΔIAP indicates a poorly compliant abdominal wall.

How do I know when abdominal wall compliance is increased?

C-abd is increased after pregnancy, previous laparoscopy or laparotomy surgery. Patients with chronic ascites have an increased C-abd after paracentesis.

Key points

- C-abd is not routinely measured in clinical practice.
- Understanding C-abd helps to understand the pathophysiological mechanisms and possible therapeutic targets.
- Decreased C-abd can be a major contributor to (secondary) IAH.

FURTHER READING

Mulier J, Dillemans B, Crombach M, Missant C, Sels A. On the abdominal pressure volume relationship. *The Internet Journal of Anesthesiology* 2009; 21(1).

Sturini E, Saporito A, Sugrue M *et al*. Respiratory variation of intra-abdominal pressure: indirect indicator of abdominal compliance? *Intensive Care Medicine* 2008; 34(9): 1632–7.

Chapter 7

Increased abdominal content

Introduction

IAP is closely related to IAV. Any change in IAV is accompanied by a change in IAP and the relationship between both is defined by C-abd.

The abdominal pressure–volume curve has two parts (see Chapter 1): a 'compensated' part where relatively large changes in volume produce only small changes in pressure and a second part, at higher volumes and pressures, in which small volume changes lead to large pressure changes.

This means that any further increase in volume in a patient with a high IAV will cause a significant increase in IAP. The reverse is true, with any decrease in IAV potentially greatly reducing IAP.

Several attempts have been made to measure, calculate or estimate IAV. Surrogate markers such as craniocaudal or anteroposterior diameter, abdominal perimeter or waist-to-hip ratio have been proposed. None of these have found to be of use to the clinician.

Measuring IAV

The abdomen includes the peritoneal cavity, the retroperitoneal space and abdominal walls. All these structures are important when considering IAP. For example, the retroperitoneal space and the abdominal wall are involved in the cause (e.g. large pelvic haematomas) and the consequences (e.g. the effects on the kidneys) of IAH.

Measuring IAV is difficult. The abdomen is irregularly shaped and its walls are not rigid. There is great variability between individuals. Several attempts to find a method to determine IAV or a clinically relevant substitute have been made.

One of these attempts considers the abdomen as a cylindrical part (the upper abdomen) on top of a conical part (the lower abdomen descending into the pelvis). In this hypothesis, the volume of the abdomen can be calculated as shown in Figure 7.1. The problem with these formulas is that there is no consensus on how to measure r or h in real patients.

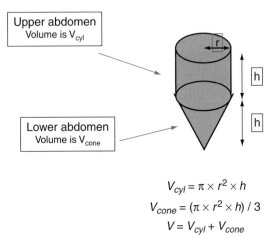

$$V_{cyl} = \pi \times r^2 \times h$$
$$V_{cone} = (\pi \times r^2 \times h) / 3$$
$$V = V_{cyl} + V_{cone}$$

Figure 7.1

Measures such as the anteroposterior, lateral or craniocaudal abdominal diameter, waist-to-hip ratio, body mass index (BMI) and others have been proposed but none has been proven to be useful.

IAV in clinical practice

Is IAV relevant?

IAH is an independent risk factor for organ dysfunction and mortality in critically ill patients. IAP is the parameter of interest and is closely linked to IAV (see Chapter 1). An increase in IAV will cause a significant increase in IAP in patients already suffering from IAH or patients with increased IAV (e.g. in the presence of pelvic haematoma, retroperitoneal inflammation caused by acute pancreatitis or retroperitoneal haematoma after ruptured aortic aneurysm, see Table 7.1).

Any decrease in IAV potentially has a significant beneficial effect on IAP. IAV is relevant to guide therapeutic interventions.

IAV and primary IAH

Primary IAH (IAH owing to an intra-abdominal cause; see Chapter 2) is often caused by increased IAV (e.g. ruptured abdominal aortic aneurysm, intra-abdominal bleeding, obstruction or pancreatitis). These conditions often require surgical intervention through laparotomy that leads to a decrease in IAV.

Table 7.1 Risk factors for the development of IAH and ACS related to increased IAV

Related to increased intra-abdominal contents
Gastroparesis
Gastric distension
Ileus
Volvulus
Colonic pseudo-obstruction (Ogilvie syndrome)
Abdominal tumour
Retroperitoneal/abdominal wall haematoma
Enteral feeding
Intra-abdominal or retroperitoneal tumour
Damage control laparotomy (packing)
Related to abdominal collections of fluid, air or blood
Liver dysfunction or cirrhosis with ascites
Abdominal infection (pancreatitis, peritonitis, abscess…)
Haemoperitoneum
Pneumoperitoneum
Laparoscopy with excessive inflation pressures
Major trauma
Peritoneal dialysis

Prophylactic open abdomen treatment can be considered when an increase in IAV is expected because of the likelihood of residual bleeding, oedema or ileus.

Examples of IAV contributing to ACS are shown in Figure 7.2A (a CT scan from a patient with obstruction causing ACS), Figure 7.2B (a CT scan from a patient with severe acute pancreatitis and retroperitoneal inflammation causing IAH) and Figure 7.2C (a CT scan from a patient with postoperative lower gastrointestinal bleeding and IAH).

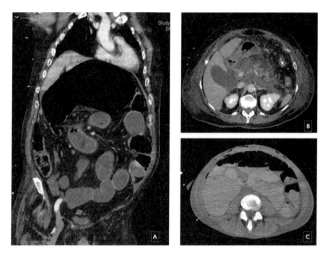

Figure 7.2

Surgery is continuously evolving with less invasive techniques being introduced, such as endovascular repair for ruptured abdominal aortic aneurysm and angiographic embolization of vessels in gastrointestinal or traumatic bleeding. These methods are successful in treating the condition for which they are used but often do not allow for IAV to be corrected. Under these conditions, IAH can develop quickly. Surgeons should consider the control of the underlying condition and its relation to IAV to avoid the risk of IAH. It may be necessary to perform a minimally invasive technique to treat the underlying cause first, but then move on early to the evacuation of intra-abdominal contents.

IAV and secondary IAH

Massive fluid resuscitation (especially using crystalloids) is a frequent cause of secondary IAH (IAH owing to an extra-abdominal cause).

Secondary IAH usually develops in patients with capillary leak syndrome caused by a systemic inflammatory event. In these patients, fluids leak out of the capillaries into the interstitial space throughout the body. In the abdominal region this leads to accumulation of oedema in the bowel, other abdominal organs and the abdominal wall. Accumulation of free peritoneal fluid and increased bowel volume due to ileus are added factors for an increased IAV.

This increased IAV and decreased C-abd combined (because of the abdominal wall oedema) can lead to secondary IAH.

Other ways in which IAV has an impact on IAH

A small increase in IAV can cause a marked increase in IAP. This can result in worsened organ dysfunction. Evacuation of even a small amount of volume can decrease IAP significantly, and bring it back into a 'safe' IAP range.

Gastric dilatation, ileus, ascites, constipation or insufflation during gastrointestinal endoscopy are all possible causes of increased IAV.

Gastrointestinal failure is one of the organ dysfunction syndromes associated with IAH. Gastric dilatation and ileus are encountered frequently in patients with IAH and will contribute to further increases in IAP. These problems should be actively sought and treated by gastroprokinetics or enemas. Free peritoneal fluid collections, however small, can be drained. Procedures leading to increased IAV such as endoscopy with insufflation should be avoided or conducted with great care, ensuring that the insufflated gas is drained out at the end of the procedure.

Key points

- IAV and IAP are interconnected: and the relationship between both is C-abd.
- In patients with IAH, a small increase in IAV can lead to aggravation of IAH.
- In the presence of IAH, a small decrease of IAV can lead to a significant decrease in IAP.
- Attempts to calculate IAV or define surrogate markers have failed to prove useful to clinicians.

FURTHER READING

De Laet IE, Ravyts M, Vidts W *et al*. Current insights in intra-abdominal hypertension and abdominal compartment syndrome: open the abdomen and keep it open! *Langenbeck's Archives of Surgery/Deutsche Gesellschaft fur Chirurgie* 2008; 393(6): 833–47.

Schachtrupp A. [Influence of volume increase on intra-abdominal pressure]. *Der Anaesthesist* 2009; 58(5): 532–6. (In German)

Chapter 8

Capillary leak and fluid resuscitation

Introduction

Capillary leak occurs during inflammation, infection and resuscitation. Capillary leak contributes to peripheral and organ oedema, pleural effusions and ascites that accompany large volume resuscitation. Capillary leak significantly contributes to the genesis of IAH and ACS.

Capillary leak represents the maladaptive, often excessive and undesirable loss of fluid and electrolytes with or without protein into the interstitium.

Capillary dynamics

The abdomen can be divided into several discrete compartments into which fluids, electrolytes and proteins are partitioned. This includes the intravascular extracellular, intravascular intracellular, extravascular intracellular and extravascular extracellular compartments. Figure 8.1 is a graphic representation of these four different fluid spaces and their relative importance. Note that the intravascular intracellular compartment is negligible in volume and often not considered.

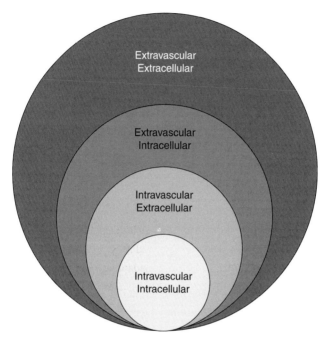

Figure 8.1

The interstitium is the extravascular extracellular compartment. The interstitium functionally behaves as a gel that allows molecule transit by diffusion. The interstitium tends to slow the free flow of fluids by maintaining the same colloid oncotic pressure in the intravascular and extravascular compartments. Under normal physiological conditions, some water and electrolytes transfer from the capillary bed to the interstitium. This is illustrated in Figure 8.2, with the capillaries acting like a leaky hosepipe. Most of the fluid

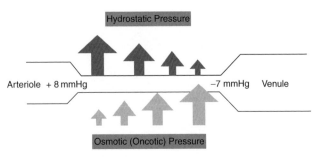

Figure 8.2

continues along the pipe but the hydrostatic pressure forces
some of water to the extravascular space. The plasma
proteins that cannot cross the capillary walls exert an osmotic
pressure that draws water back into the capillaries. This oncotic
force is greater than the hydrostatic pressure at the venous
end of the capillaries. The net effect at the arteriolar site is
+8 mmHg and forces fluids into the interstitium; the net
pressure at the venous site is −7 mmHg and drives fluids back
into the capillaries. This results in about 20 litres of water
being transferred out and about 16 litres being reabsorbed
every day.

The capillary surface properties determine the filtration
coefficient. A high value indicates a capillary that is highly
permeable to water and a low value indicates the opposite. The
permeability factor is often expressed as the 'hydraulic
conductivity' of the capillary wall, in which the surface area is
considered.

Capillary injuries generally increase the filtration coefficient.
Increases in interstitial water and solute volume occur when the

Table 8.1 Factors influencing fluid movement across the capillary bed

Increases in the hydrostatic gradient between the capillary and interstitial space	Decreases in the oncotic gradient between the capillary and interstitial space
Increased capillary hydrostatic pressure	*Decreased capillary oncotic pressure*
Fluid overload	Malnutrition
Arterial vasodilatation	Dilution secondary to crystalloid plasma volume expansion
Venous obstruction	
Decreased interstitial hydrostatic pressure	*Increased interstitial oncotic pressure*
Negative pressure pulmonary oedema	Capillary protein leak

normal balance of forces is disturbed, as in the conditions described in Table 8.1.

Capillary leak in the critically ill patient

Increases in hydrostatic pressure and decreases in vascular colloid oncotic pressure will occur in the critically ill patient because of plasma volume expansion, acute hypoproteinemia secondary to dilution, pre-existing or acquired severe protein and calorie deficiencies.

These effects are exacerbated by the capillary leak associated with inflammation or infection. Tight junctions between capillary endothelial cells are loosened during these pathophysiological processes and functional holes appear in the capillary wall, causing water, electrolytes and protein to flow from the vascular to the interstitial space.

Once shock is established, sympathetically driven vasoconstriction diverts blood to perfuse the heart and brain preferentially. This flow redistribution leads to hypoperfusion of peripheral tissues. If not corrected, cellular hypoxia leads to cell death.

Simultaneously, macrophages, monocytes, mast cells, platelets and endothelial cells produce a multitude of small molecules (cytokines) that will directly or indirectly activate the coagulation and complement cascades, trigger nitric oxide synthesis and release, activate platelet-activating factor and modulate biosynthesis of prostaglandins and leukotrienes. These activities alter the pre-capillary arteriolar tone and tissue perfusion. Protein complements C3a and C5a contribute directly to the release of additional cytokines and cause vasodilatation and increased vascular permeability.

Neutrophils recruited during the tissue hypoperfusion are primed to generate toxic oxygen metabolites. These inflammatory moieties directly damage lipid membranes and interstitial enzyme complexes, including matrix metalloproteinases.

This process is interrupted by fluid resuscitation. Plasma volume expansion seeks to restore both macrocirculatory and microcirculatory flow. As flow returns to hypoperfused tissues, it brings a large amount of oxygen. All the processes are amplified and the lipid and enzyme destruction alters the barrier between the vascular and interstitial compartments. Heparan sulfate is released, under the influences of oxidative damage. Some cells undergo apoptotic death regardless of intervention; other cells will either survive or die depending on the balance between salutary and deleterious effects of resuscitation. The cumulative effect promotes capillary leak.

During capillary leak, plasma volume expansion with crystalloid solutions increases extravascular fluid accumulation as the vascular oncotic pressure is further decreased by dilution.

Peripheral oedema, visceral organ oedema and ascites develop across the abdominal cavity. Pleural effusion builds up in the thorax.

Aggressive fluid resuscitation, as suggested by the Early Goal Directed Therapy paradigm, may exacerbate the issue of capillary leak syndrome. This may lead to rapid ascites formation and resulting likelihood of secondary IAH and ACS, as shown in Figure 8.3.

Secondary IAH and ACS are increasingly identified in the context of acute infections, such as pneumonia and septic shock, treated with significant plasma volume expansion.

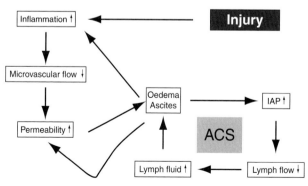

Figure 8.3

Increased awareness of these issues resulting from aggressive resuscitation is likely to increase the clinical recognition of IAH and its consequences.

IAP and the three hits model of shock

In 1942, Cuthbertson introduced the concept of a dual metabolic response to bodily injury.

Table 8.2 summarizes the three hits models.

The ebb phase

The ebb phase represents a distributive shock characterized by arterial vasodilatation and transcapillary albumin leakage

Table 8.2 Hit models of shock

	First hit	Second hit	Third hit
Cause	Inflammatory insult	Ischaemia–reperfusion	Global increased permeability syndrome
Phase	Ebb	Flow	No flow
Fluids	Life-saving	Biomarker of illness	Toxic
Monitoring	Functional, haemodynamic	Organ function	Perfusion
Treatment	Early adequate goal directed fluid management	Late conservative fluid management	Late goal directed fluid removal
Fluid balance	Positive	Neutral	Negative

abating plasma oncotic pressure, and is the response to the initial proinflammatory cytokines and stress hormones. Arterial vascular collapse, microcirculatory dysfunction and secondary interstitial oedema lead to systemic hypoperfusion and regional impaired tissue use of oxygen. Compensatory neuroendocrine reflexes and potential renal dysfunction cause sodium and water retention, leading to a positive fluid balance.

The flow phase

Patients overcoming shock attain homeostasis of proinflammatory and anti-inflammatory mediators within 3 days. Subsequent haemodynamic stabilization and restoration of plasma oncotic pressure start the *flow phase* with resumption of diuresis and mobilization of extravascular fluid resulting in negative fluid balances.

The global increased permeability syndrome

The global increased permeability syndrome (GIPS) is characterized by high capillary leak index (expressed as C-reactive protein over albumin ratio), excess interstitial fluid and persistent high extravascular lung water (EVLW), inability to refrain giving more fluid to the patient as it is clinically indicated and progressive organ failure. GIPS represents a 'third hit' following acute injury with progression to multi-organ failure (MOF).

Capillary leaks and impaired flow phase mean that overzealous administration of fluids in GIPS causes gross fluid overload and tissue oedema. Interstitial oedema raises the pressure in all major body compartments: head, chest, abdomen and extremities. Venous resistance of organs enclosed in compartments increases and perfusion pressure decreases. This progresses to organ failure.

All compartments interact and reciprocally transmit pressures, supporting the notion of a polycompartment syndrome.

The abdomen plays a central role in GIPS and the polycompartment syndrome and positive fluid balances are a known risk factor for secondary IAH. Secondary IAH is associated with deleterious effects on other compartments and organ functions.

Renal function in particular is strongly affected by IAH. Furthermore, renal interstitial oedema in absence of IAH may impair renal function. Therefore, fluid overload leading to IAH and associated renal dysfunction may counteract its own resolution. Figure 8.4 illustrates the vicious circle to which this may lead.

Adverse effects of capillary leak are particularly pronounced in the lungs, and monitoring of EVLW is suggested as a possible tool to guide fluid management. A high EVLW indicates a state of capillary leakage, associated with higher severity of illness and mortality. EVLW has a prognostic value as a reflection of the extent of capillary leakage, rather than as a quantification of lung function impairment by lung water.

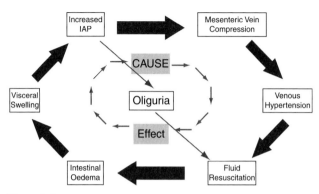

Figure 8.4

This has direct consequences on fluid management in the critically ill patient with IAH. Patients at risk of GIPS require restrictive fluid strategies and fluid removal guided by extended haemodynamic monitoring, including EVLW measurements. Restrictive fluid management may require a greater use of vasopressor therapy, resuscitation with hyperoncotic solutions (e.g. albumin 20%) and early initiation of diuretics and renal replacement therapy.

Figure 8.5 illustrates the GIPS and its relation to the three hits theory.

Table 8.3 lists the consequences of fluid overload.

Table 8.4 lists the risk factors for the development of IAH and ACS in the context of capillary leaks.

When it starts to get better (day 3)

The dual response to acute inflammatory insult is characterized by a turning point on day 3. Homeostasis of cytokines allows

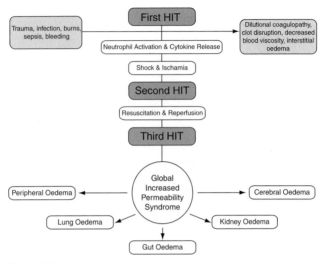

Figure 8.5

initiation of correction of the microcirculatory disruptions and 'closure' of the capillary leaks. Microcirculatory blood flow seems to normalize on day 3 in patients with abdominal sepsis.

Key points

- Capillary leak is a result of the inflammatory response and its diverse triggers, including ischaemia–reperfusion.
- Plasma volume expansion to correct hypoperfusion predictably results in extravascular movement of water, electrolytes and proteins.

Table 8.3 Consequences of capillary leaks and fluid overload

System	Effect
Central nervous system	Cerebral oedema increases
	Impaired cognition
	Delirium
	Intracranial pressure increases
	Cerebral perfusion pressure decreases
	Intraocular pressure increases
	Intracranial hypertension
Respiratory system	Pulmonary oedema
	Impaired gas exchange
	Hypercarbia
	PaO_2 and PaO_2/FiO_2 decrease
	Extravascular lung water increases
	Prolonged ventilation
	Difficult weaning
	Increased work of breathing
Renal system	Renal interstitial oedema
	Renal venous pressure increases
	Renal blood flow decreases
	Interstitial pressure increases
	Glomerular filtration rate decreases
	Uraemia
	Renal vascular resistance increases
	Salt retention increases
	Water retention increases
	Renal compartment syndrome
Abdominal wall	Tissue oedema increases
	Lymphatic drainage decreases
	Microcirculation decreases

Table 8.3 (cont.)

System	Effect
	Poor wound healing
	Wound infection increases
	Pressure ulcers
Endocrine system	Release of cytokines
Gastrointestinal system	Gut oedema increases
	Malabsorption
	Ileus
	Abdominal perfusion pressure decreases
	Bowel contractility decreases
	IAP increases and incidence of IAH and ACS increase
	Successful enteral feeding decreases
	Intestinal permeability increases
	Bacterial translocation increases
Hepatic system	Hepatic congestion
	Impaired synthetic function
	Cholestasis
	Impaired cytochrome P450 activty
	Hepatic compartment syndrome
Cardiovascular system	Myocardial oedema
	Conduction disturbances
	Impaired contractility
	Diastolic dysfunction

- Plasma volume expansion in the context of GIPS can lead to IAH, and sometimes ACS.
- A variety of strategies are available to the clinician to reduce the volume of fluids used during resuscitation and this may affect the occurrence of IAH.

Table 8.4 Risk factors for the development of IAH and ACS

In the context of capillary leak and fluid resuscitation

Acidosis (pH below 7.2)

Hypothermia (core temperature below 33°C)

Coagulopathy [platelet count below 50 000/mm^3 or an activated partial
    thromboplastin time (APTT) greater than twice normal or a prothrombin time
    (PTT) below 50% or an international standardized ratio (INR) greater than 1.5]

Polytransfusion/trauma (>10 units of packed red cells/24 hours)

Sepsis

Severe sepsis or bacteraemia

Septic shock

Massive fluid resuscitation (3–5 L of colloid or >10 L of crystalloid/24 hours with
    capillary leak and positive fluid balance)

Major burns

FURTHER READING

Cordemans C, De laet I, Van Regenmortel N *et al.* Fluid
    management in critically ill patients: The role of
    extravascular lung water, abdominal hypertension, capillary
    leak and fluid balance. *Annals of Intensive Care* 2012; 2
    (Suppl. 1): S1.

Cuthbertson DP. Post-shock metabolic response. *Lancet*
    1942; 239: 433–7.

Fishel RS, Chandrakanth A, Barbul B. Vessel injury and
    capillary leak. *Critical Care Medicine* 2003; 31(8): S502–11.

Matsuda N, Hattori Y. Vascular biology in sepsis:
    pathophysiological and therapeutic significance of vascular
    dysfunction. *Journal of Smooth Muscle Research* 2007; 43
    (4): 117–37.

Maxwell RA, Fabian TC, Croce MA, Davis KA.
Secondary abdominal compartment syndrome: an
underappreciated manifestation of severe hemorrhagic
shock. *Journal of Trauma* 1999; 47(6):
995–9.

Specific conditions: when to worry more?

Chapter 9

Pancreatitis

Introduction

IAH is an important contributor to early organ dysfunction in severe acute pancreatitis, and is associated with pancreatic necrosis. Up to 80% of patients with severe acute pancreatitis will develop IAH. ACS is observed in 30% of these patients. Prompt recognition, prevention of IAH and treatment of the ACS are essential to avoid irreversible deterioration.

Why and when do patients with severe acute pancreatitis develop IAH and ACS?

IAH can be present at admission or occur shortly thereafter, with ACS developing mostly within the first few days. IAH is caused by the inflammatory process causing retroperitoneal oedema, fluid retention, ascites, ileus and decreasing abdominal wall compliance. Aggressive fluid resuscitation will contribute to IAH. Figure 9.1 shows an abdominal CT scan obtained early after admission of a patient with pancreatitis. Retroperitoneal inflammation and fluid collections are present.

IAH and ACS can appear later, 1 or more weeks after initial presentation. This late appearance is often associated with local

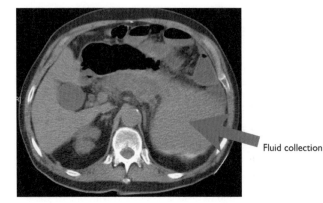

Fluid collection

Figure 9.1

pancreatic complications such as bleeding or infected peripancreatic necrosis.

Consequences of IAH and ACS in the patient with severe acute pancreatitis

IAH and ACS are associated with impaired organ dysfunction, especially of the cardiovascular, respiratory and renal systems. It can be difficult to differentiate between the systemic inflammatory response syndrome (SIRS) of the pancreatitis process itself and the effects of ACS. Respiratory insufficiency in the non-ventilated patient or increased ventilatory issues in ventilated patients should raise the possibility of IAH or ACS. Elevated hemidiaphragms and bilateral pleural effusions may be observed. Oliguria is a common feature and additional fluid loading will further exacerbate IAH or ACS.

The mortality rate in patients with severe acute pancreatitis developing ACS is 50–75% (if not treated). Early mortality in severe acute pancreatitis is often related to unrecognized ACS.

Diagnosis of IAH and ACS in the patient with severe acute pancreatitis

IAH and ACS is considered to be present in all patients with severe acute pancreatitis until proven otherwise. IAH cannot reliably be diagnosed clinically and IAP measurement is mandatory in all patients admitted with severe acute pancreatitis. The IAP should be measured regularly (every 2–4 hours when using intermittent IAP measurement). An IAP greater than 20 mmHg is diagnostic and requires treatment.

Recognizing IAH before ACS develops is essential. A practical algorithm is suggested in Figure 9.2.

Prevention of IAH and ACS in the patient with severe acute pancreatitis

The progression from IAH to ACS will usually take 1–2 days but may be faster. The recognition and treatment of IAH is required to prevent ACS. Aside from standard medical management (see Section 5), percutaneous drainage of abdominal fluid collections may be useful in the context of severe acute pancreatitis. It is advised that crystalloids are used judiciously in patients with impending ACS.

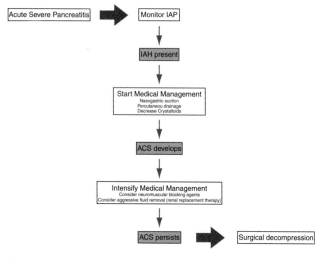

Figure 9.2

Treatment of IAH and ACS in the patient with severe acute pancreatitis

Surgery

Surgery is not required in all patients. Non-surgical and percutaneous interventions should be tried first (see Table 9.1).

Surgical decompression should be considered when non-surgical measures have failed to decrease IAP and improve respiratory and cardiovascular function. Urine output will resume early when medical interventions have successfully decreased IAP. Renal dysfunction (independent

Table 9.1 Non-surgical decompression to decrease IAH in severe acute pancreatitis

Decompression with a nasogastric drainage tube
Short-term use of neuromuscular blockers
Removal of excess fluid by diuretics
Removal of excess fluid with extracorporeal techniques
Ultrasound-guided percutaneous drainage of ascites

of urine output) will recover slowly, especially after prolonged IAH.

Surgical decompression can be achieved with a midline laparotomy where all layers (skin, fascia, peritoneum) are divided through a vertical midline incision extending from the sternum to the pubis. This procedure requires temporary cover of the open wound. Preference is given to dressings that create a negative pressure in the abdomen and prevent the retraction of the wound edges. Dressing changes are needed every 2–3 days and can be done either in the operating room or the intensive care unit. Time to close should be guided by IAP measurements.

Other methods include bilateral incisions a few centimetres below the costal margins or three short horizontal skin incisions to perform a subcutaneous linea alba fasciotomy (SLAF). With a SLAF, the peritoneum is left intact and it may be less effective than other methods. The procedure should be tailored to the patient and SLAF can be an elegant first step to reduce IAP. Several methods can be used in succession. Endoscope-guided retroperitoneal techniques have been suggested.

Regardless of the surgical decompression method it is important to continue to measure IAP postoperatively to recognize recurrent ACS.

Feeding

Studies have shown that early enteral nutrition is beneficial in patients with acute pancreatitis. Most patients did not have organ dysfunction, and the impact on and of IAH has not been studied.

Reduction of enteral feeding to 20 mL/h should be considered when IAH develops. Enteral nutrition should be stopped if IAH evolves into ACS.

When can the clinician stop considering IAH in patients with severe acute pancreatitis?

Discharge from ICU is the time when you can stop thinking of IAH in patients with severe acute pancreatitis. Note that complications associated with IAH can manifest weeks later, linked to infection or bleeding. Any new or recurrent organ dysfunction may suggest IAH.

Key points

- IAH and ACS are common in severe acute pancreatitis.
- Always suspect IAH in severe acute pancreatitis and measure IAP regularly.
- Do not allow IAP greater than 20 mmHg.

- Try non-surgical decompression measures first but do not hesitate to resort to surgical decompression at an early stage.

FURTHER READING

De Waele JJ, Hoste E, Blot SI *et al.* Intra-abdominal hypertension in patients with severe acute pancreatitis. *Critical Care* 2005; 9: R452–7.

Chapter 10

Children

Introduction

Published definitions of IAH and ACS are related to standardized IAP monitoring, and these facilitate research and improve patient care. These definitions and standard techniques are not all directly applicable to children.

IAP in children

Normal values of IAP in children

Normal IAP in spontaneously breathing children is reported to be 0 mmHg or subatmospheric. Normal IAP in mechanically ventilated children is reported to be 7 ± 3 mmHg.

Measurement of IAP in children.

IAP can be monitored in children by various techniques; the most common method is intermittent measurement via the bladder. Continuous bladder pressure monitoring (see Chapter 4) is difficult in children as it relies on three-way urethral catheters which are too large.

Accurate readings require a standardized volume of fluid to be instilled into the bladder. Some suggest instilling 1 mL/kg of fluid, with a maximum of 20 mL. Volumes of 5 mL or even as low as 3 mL are used.

Factors that affect accurate IAP readings are similar to those in adults (see Chapter 5) except that the BMI does not seem to be important in children.

Monitoring variability in IAP across time and integrating IAP values with other vital signs is especially important in children.

No commercial IAP monitoring kits are specifically designed for use in children, but the AbViser® Neonate adaptor (AbViser Medical, USA, recently acquired by ConvaTec Medical, USA) allows the use of feeding tubes as improvised urethral catheters in smaller infants (Figure 10.1).

Accurate IAP readings can be affected by the factors detailed in Chapter 5. Abdominal muscle contractions that occur when a child is crying will affect IAP readings. Infants use their abdominal muscles to breathe and usually have a high

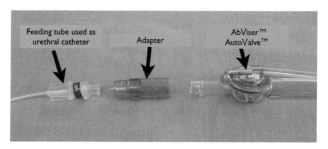

Figure 10.1

respiratory rate. This renders the acquisition of measurements at end-expiration challenging. For this reason, a child with respiratory distress may present with erroneously high IAP readings. In some circumstances it may be necessary to sedate or paralyse a child to obtain appropriate measures.

In the absence of outcome studies in children, practical goals include lowering the IAP to less than 10 mmHg and keeping the abdominal perfusion pressure above 35 mmHg in infants and up to 60 mmHg or greater in larger children.

Outcomes of IAP in children

Evidence of organ damage has been reported to occur with IAP greater than 10 mmHg. ACS occurs in children at a lower IAP.

IAP, IAH and ACS are independent predictors of mortality in children. Conversely, the Paediatric Risk of Mortality (PRISM) III score has been associated with increased risk for IAH when the score is greater or equal to 17.

IAH and ACS in children

Diagnosis of IAH and ACS in children

Recognition of IAH in children requires a high index of clinical suspicion. The value of IAP at which organ damage occurs varies according to premorbid conditions, underlying causal factors and mean arterial blood pressure. At this undefined critical pressure, reduction in microcirculatory

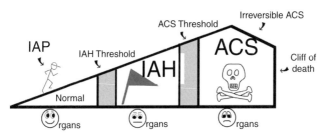

Figure 10.2

blood flow occurs, and the development of organ dysfunction begins.

The astute clinician will not disregard a diagnosis of ACS because the IAP has not reached 20 mmHg. The exact IAP at which IAH becomes ACS is not known. Figure 10.2 illustrates how IAP critical value can vary. In children, any elevation in IAP that is associated with a new organ dysfunction is ACS unless proven otherwise.

IAH has been reported in a wide variety of diseases in the medical and surgical paediatric population (Table 10.1).

Management of IAH and ACS in children

The management of ACS in children is dependent upon, and directed toward, the etiology of the underlying problem.

The ideal treatment for ACS depends on its early recognition. Prevention of ACS by constant measurement of IAH is essential.

Spring-loaded Silastic silos are used in the management of gastroschisis. Biological membranes can be used to cover exposed viscera of ruptured omphaloceles.

Table 10.1 Conditions associated with increased risk for ACS in children

Primary ACS	Secondary ACS
Gastroschisis	Aggressive fluid resuscitation
Omphalocele	Sepsis/capillary leak syndrome
Necrotizing enterocolitis	Multiple transfusions of blood products
Abdominal tumours	Multiple trauma
Intra-abdominal infections, e.g. appendicitis, peritonitis, toxic megacolon	Hypothermia
Bowel obstruction, ischaemia or infarction	Failed Fontan procedure/heart failure with increased venous pressure
Abdominal trauma/haemorrhage	Renal failure
Complications of abdominal surgery	Extracorporeal membrane oxygenation
Ascites	Burns
Disproportionate solid organ transplant	Bone marrow transplant
Ileus, aganglionosis, constipation	

ACS requires expeditious decompression. This can be achieved by paracentesis or a peritoneal drain in cases of fluid accumulation being the cause of IAH. ACS caused by visceral swelling requires surgical decompression by laparotomy and temporary abdominal closure with a vacuum pack, prosthetic mesh, Wittmann patch or vacuum-assisted closure system. ACS can recur despite temporary abdominal closure, and continued monitoring is essential. Medical management must continue alongside surgical release.

Key points

- Normal IAP in mechanically ventilated children is about 7 mmHg.
- Critical values of IAP that suggest IAH and ACS are lower in children.
- In children, IAP greater than 10 mmHg should be considered to be IAH.
- IAP above 10 mmHg associated with new organ dysfunction is ACS in children until proven otherwise.
- Abdominal breathing in children may result in erroneous IAP readings.

FURTHER READING

Ejike JC, Bahjri K, Mathur M. What is normal intra-abdominal pressure in critically ill children and how should we measure it? *Critical Care Medicine* 2008; 36: 2157–62.

Ejike JC, Humbert S, Bahjri K, Mathur M. Outcomes of children with abdominal compartment syndrome. *Acta Clinica Belgica Supplement* 2007; 1: 141–8.

Ejike JC, Kadry J, Bahjri K, Mathur M. Semi-recumbent position and body mass percentiles: effects on intra-abdominal pressure measurements in critically ill children. *Intensive Care Medicine* 2010; 36(2): 329–35.

Chapter **11**

Trauma

Introduction

Occurrence of ACS is not limited to abdominal trauma patients. Secondary ACS can be a frequent complication in severely injured patients if IAH is not prevented. All patients sustaining severe trauma, irrespective of its location, are at risk of developing IAH and ACS. Prevention of secondary ACS is possible by the application of 'damage control' surgery, judicious fluid resuscitation and adherence to specific transfusion protocols.

In patients requiring 'damage control' surgery, leaving the abdomen open is a key element in preventing ACS. When ACS develops in trauma patients, early decompression is advised. After decompression, non-surgical measures will allow early abdominal closure.

Organ dysfunction is a marker of development of IAH and ACS.

Types of ACS in trauma patients

Both primary and secondary ACS are commonly seen in trauma patients.

The usual presentation of primary ACS is severe abdominal trauma requiring 'damage control' laparotomy with (or without) packing and abdominal closure. While the abdominal trauma is the direct cause, mechanisms leading to secondary ACS such as fluid resuscitation contribute to further deterioration.

All types of extra-abdominal trauma can lead to secondary ACS. Secondary ACS usually develops later than primary ACS but should be considered at any time if organ dysfunction develops. This may happen within the first 12 hours after injury, and IAP monitoring is always indicated in severely injured patients.

Incidence

The incidence of IAH and ACS in trauma patients is decreasing rapidly as centres have embraced these concepts and apply strategies that avoid the occurrence of both primary and secondary ACS. A few years ago, the incidence of ACS was as high as 40% with high mortality rates. It has reduced dramatically in recent years. The occurrence of ACS in trauma patients is now considered an indicator of suboptimal trauma care.

The 'bloody' vicious circle and IAH

The 'bloody vicious cycle' or 'lethal triad' of trauma patients is the combination of coagulopathy, hypothermia and acidosis. These three factors contribute to ongoing blood loss from the injured body. Ischaemia/reperfusion injury occurs at the initiation of resuscitation.

Early control of blood losses and restoration of the coagulation capabilities of the blood are important in avoiding this lethal triad. Resulting oedema (inside and outside the abdominal cavity) will result in IAH. Strategies aimed at preventing this lethal triad will effectively prevent ACS. 'Damage control' surgery aims at early and rapid control of blood loss. Prophylactic open abdomen management is an early step. Rapid transfer of the patient to an intensive care unit to correct acidosis, hypothermia and coagulopathy is essential. Definitive repair of non-life-threatening injuries can be delayed to a later stage.

It is often difficult to distinguish ACS from shock, continuous bleeding and related inflammatory responses. To help differentiate between these, IAP measurement is required early in trauma patients.

Predicting factors of IAH in the trauma patient are shown in Table 11.1.

Table 11.1 Predictors of ACS in trauma patients

Primary ACS	Secondary ACS
Temperature <34°C	Administration of >7.5 L of crystalloids before ICU admission
Haemoglobin <8 g/dL	No indication for life-saving surgical intervention
Base deficit >8 mmol/L	Relatively low urine output (<50 mL/h)
Administration of >3 L of crystalloids	Poor intestinal perfusion measured by gastric tonometry
Transfusion of ≥3 units of red cells	
Need for emergency surgery	

Conservative management of the patient with abdominal trauma

Conservative management of the trauma patient does not mitigate the risk of IAH and ACS. Patients may have lost considerable amounts of blood in the peritoneum, and other factors (such as oedema formation due to shock from extra-abdominal injuries or ileus) may contribute to the development of IAH. These mechanisms explain why IAH can happen in patients treated with angiographic embolization.

Laparotomy is the definitive treatment option if residual bleeding from the initial injury persists. Reports of successful percutaneous drainage using large bore catheters are encouraging.

Similar to patients with severe acute pancreatitis, trauma patients who develop secondary ACS may benefit from a subcutaneous linea alba fasciotomy (SLAF). This is an attractive alternative in patients who did not require an initial abdominal surgical intervention.

IAH in the patient with an open abdomen

The risk for ACS in patients with an open abdomen is low but new issues (such as bleeding) may lead to an increase in IAP. A midline laparotomy may be inadequate (too small) to decompress the abdomen fully.

Moreover, IAP can decrease after abdominal decompression but still remain above the threshold for continued damage to various organ systems. Medical strategies to decrease IAP further are important to reverse organ dysfunction. An open abdomen is just one element in the treatment, and does not preclude the development of IAH and ACS.

The abdomen should remain open as long as this benefits the patient, but attempts should be made to close the abdomen early. A fine balance is required. Continued IAP measurement is indicated to help make the right decision.

Key points

- IAH and ACS can occur both in abdominal trauma and extra-abdominal trauma patients.
- Patients at risk for IAH should be identified at an early stage of their treatment.
- IAP must be measured regularly in all severely injured patients irrespective of the site of injury.
- Early bleeding control and avoiding massive transfusion are key elements in preventing IAH in trauma patients.
- Open abdomen treatment should be applied liberally in patients at risk.
- The use of medical management strategies to reduce IAP will facilitate early closure of the abdomen, and avoid complications related to open abdomen treatment.

FURTHER READING

Ball CG, Kirkpatrick AW, McBeth P. The secondary abdominal compartment syndrome: not just another post-traumatic complication. *Canadian Journal of Surgery* 2008; 51: 399–405.

Cheatham ML, Safcsak K. Is the evolving management of intra-abdominal hypertension and abdominal compartment syndrome improving survival? *Critical Care Medicine* 2010; 38: 402–7.

Rizoli S, Mamtani A, Scarpelini S, Kirkpatrick AW. Abdominal compartment syndrome in trauma resuscitation. *Current Opinion in Anaesthesiology* 2010; 23: 251–7.

Chapter **12**

Burns

Introduction

Severe burn patients develop IAH/ACS within 48 hours. The increase in capillary permeability contributes to extensive oedema formation and intraperitoneal accumulation of fluid. Gut oedema and fluid translocation is worsened by venous hypertension caused by an elevated IAP.

Figure 12.1 shows the relationship between the resuscitation fluid volume received within the first 24 hours of the insult, the percentage of the total body surface area that has been burned and ACS.

Secondary ACS in burn patients generally occurs within 48 hours of the injury, during the initial resuscitation period. The risk decreases substantially when the patient reaches the 'diuretic phase'. The risk for IAH/ACS increases again if the patient develops sepsis.

Incidence

The incidence of IAH depends on the severity of the burn injury. The risk of ACS is directly related to the burned area.

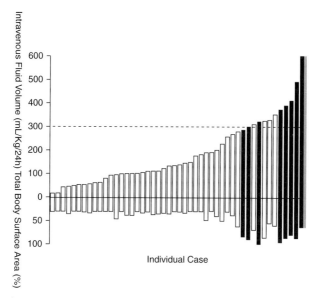

Figure 12.1

Consequences of IAH in the patient with severe burns

IAH is associated with impaired organ dysfunction, including the cardiovascular, respiratory and renal systems. In severe burn patients, the kidneys become vulnerable and preserving renal function is particularly important. ACS alone, or when associated with its surgical treatment, increases the risk of multiple organ dysfunction, including acute lung injury. The mortality rate of patients developing ACS is 50–80%, even when treated.

Monitoring IAP in the burn patient

IAH/ACS should be considered in all patients with severe
burns. IAP measurement should be performed every 2–4 hours
throughout the resuscitation period in burn patients with more
than 20% of their body area affected.

IAH/ACS might occur in patients without circumferential
third degree burn of their trunk. Figure 12.2 shows a patient
with a tense abdomen despite normal elasticity of the
abdominal wall. Measurement of the IAP revealed a pressure
of 60 mmHg.

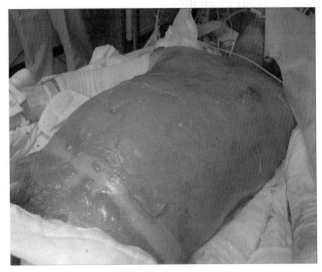

Figure 12.2

IAH prevention in the burn patient

Key to the prevention of ACS is the early recognition and treatment of IAH. Avoiding over-resuscitation is important, because this is an element in the development of secondary ACS. Percutaneous drainage of any abdominal fluid collection may reduce IAP.

The choice of resuscitation fluid appears to be important. Randomized studies have shown that hypertonic lactated saline or plasma-based resuscitation requires a lower volume of fluids, and these are associated with a lower risk of development of IAH and ACS.

Urine output as an indicator during resuscitation of the burn patient

The urine output is often cited as an easy indicator to use during resuscitation of the burn patient. Although this is true for some patients, oliguria will no longer be caused by fluid depletion when IAH and ACS develop. In this situation, increasing resuscitation volumes will worsen the problem. Advanced haemodynamic monitoring is indicated to direct fluid resuscitation, and interventions to reduce IAP should be undertaken early.

Treatment of IAH in the burn patient

Non-surgical and percutaneous interventions should be applied before surgical decompression is considered. Nasogastric decompression, the use of neuromuscular blockers and the removal of excess fluid by ultrasound-guided percutaneous drainage of ascites are simple and effective methods to reduce IAP.

Escharotomy of the trunk should be performed, especially in the presence of third degree burns.

Midline laparotomy may make wound management more difficult in abdominal burn patients, yet it remains very effective in reducing IAP.

Regardless of surgical decompression, it is important to continue to measure the IAP postoperatively to recognize recurrent ACS. The open abdomen after laparotomy requires a temporary abdominal closure technique. The presence of abdominal burns may pose specific challenges to the management of the open abdomen.

Key points

- IAH will develop in most, if not all, severely burned patients.
- Always suspect IAH and measure the IAP regularly in the resuscitation period.
- Escharotomy can dramatically reduce IAP in case of abdominal burns.
- Decompression laparotomy is a definitive therapy, but wound maintenance and infection control are difficult.

FURTHER READING

Kirkpatrick AW, Ball CG, Nickerson D *et al*. Intra-abdominal hypertension and the abdominal compartment syndrome in burn patients. *World Journal of Surgery* 2009; 33: 1142–9.

Oda J, Yamashita K, Inoue T *et al.* Resuscitation fluid volume and abdominal compartment syndrome in patients with major burns. *Burns* 2006; 32: 151–4.

Oda J, Yamashita K, Inoue T *et al.* Acute lung injury and multiple organ dysfunction syndrome secondary to intra-abdominal hypertension and abdominal decompression in extensively burned patients. *Journal of Trauma* 2007; 62: 1365–9.

Chapter 13

Obesity

Introduction

Obesity is defined as a BMI of 30 kg/m^2 or greater.

Obesity is becoming an endemic problem, with many nations reporting increased BMI in their population.

Numerous studies have demonstrated a link between obesity and elevated IAP. Mean IAP in morbidly obese subjects (BMI greater than 35 kg/m^2) has been reported to be around 9 mmHg. This can be compared to the mean IAP in smaller size women, measured at 0 mmHg. The difference is explained by an unproven direct mass effect caused by intra-abdominal adipose tissue.

Elevated IAP might be the cause of obesity-related comorbidities, such as hypertension, pseudotumour cerebri, pulmonary complications, gastro-oesophageal reflux disease and abdominal wall hernia.

Normal values of IAP in obese patients

The baseline IAP is higher in obese patients and any change in IAP will impact on organ function. A number of chronic ailments are attributed to the chronic elevated IAP, but it appears that a higher absolute level of IAP may be required in morbidly obese patients to cause acute organ dysfunction.

IAP and chronic morbidity in the obese patient

Systemic hypertension

An acute increase in IAP is associated with an increase in central venous pressure and systemic vascular resistance, and a decrease in venous return, cardiac output, visceral blood flow and renal blood flow.

Chronic IAP is indirectly associated with hypertension as a normal IAP appears to offer a protective effect against systemic hypertension. The pathogenesis is unknown, and remains controversial.

Pseudotumour cerebri

Morbidly obese individuals have significantly higher IAP and a higher prevalence of pseudotumour cerebri. An acute increase of IAP to 25 mmHg above baseline causes a significant increase in intracranial pressure in animal models. Cerebral venous outflow becomes obstructed owing to increased pleural and associated thoracic pressures.

Respiratory morbidity

Morbidly obese individuals are at a higher risk of respiratory complications. Both forced expiratory volume and forced vital capacity are inversely correlated to IAP, thereby suggesting that an elevated IAP may result in pulmonary restrictive disorders.

Gastro-oesophageal reflux

Gastro-oesophageal reflux disease is prevalent among the morbidly obese. In IAH, the resistance gradient between the stomach and the gastro-oesophageal junction should be higher in the obese subject. However, gastro-oesophageal reflux happens at a lower mean IAP in morbidly obese patients.

Incisional hernia

Chronic IAH has been postulated to cause incisional hernias. No correlation between IAP and the presence of an incisional hernia has, however, been proven.

Specifics of IAP management in the obese patient

There are no 'specifics' in the management of IAP in the obese patient. Abdominal decompression will be more challenging and difficult to achieve, mainly for practical reasons.

Key points

- IAP in the morbidly obese patient is abnormally elevated.
- Acute elevations in IAP have similar effects in obese patients, but the threshold before organ dysfunction develops may be higher.

- Chronic elevations in IAP may, in part, be responsible for the pathogenesis of obesity-related conditions.

FURTHER READING

Lambert DM, Marceau S, Forse RA. Intra-abdominal pressure in the morbidly obese. *Obesity Surgery* 2005; 15: 1225–32.
Varela JE, Hinojosa M, Nguyen N. Correlations between intra-abdominal pressure and obesity-related co-morbidities. *Surgery for Obesity and Related Diseases* 2009; 5: 524–8.

Chapter 14

Pregnancy and others

Introduction

Many common clinical conditions and procedures, e.g. pregnancy, obesity, peritoneal dialysis, pneumoperitoneum, prone positioning and application of end-expiratory positive pressure, are associated with elevated IAP.

Some of these conditions present with symptoms concordant with ACS, but the presence of these symptoms is not solely caused by elevated IAP.

Pregnancy and IAP

The uterus occupies a major part of the abdominal cavity during the second and third trimesters of pregnancy. Breathlessness and decrease in blood pressure are observed in the supine parturient ('supine hypotension syndrome'). These symptoms are caused by the disruption of diaphragmatic motions and the compression of the inferior vena cava. These symptoms are alleviated in the lateral, sitting or standing positions.

Surprisingly, IAP is usually not elevated in the normal pregnant woman.

The abdominal wall is slowly stretched under hormonal influences and increases its compliance, reducing the potential for an increase in IAP caused by the expanding uterus.

If IAP increases for other reasons, such as pneumoperitoneum at laparoscopy, it can severely compromise the perfusion of the uterus and the fetus.

Peritoneal dialysis and IAP

IAP may be markedly increased during peritoneal dialysis, when a significant amount of dialysis fluid, up to 4 L in an adult, is poured into the peritoneal cavity.

This increase in IAP has been shown to lead to decreased cardiac output and increased pulmonary artery pressures. This is why peritoneal dialysis is not recommended in the intensive care patient. It may explain, in part, the higher mortality rates observed in patients receiving peritoneal dialysis rather than continuous veno-venous haemofiltration.

If patients are established and receive peritoneal dialysis on a regular basis, blood pressures and cardiac index might remain unchanged despite a twofold increase in IAP. This is, however, controversial. High IAP has been identified as a risk factor for abdominal wall complications in patients on chronic ambulatory peritoneal dialysis (CAPD). Recent studies therefore advocate limiting the filling pressures during CAPD to 14 mmHg.

Peritoneal dialysis is usually better tolerated in children and it is still a common procedure in infants and children who develop acute renal failure after cardiac surgery.

IAP during iatrogenic pneumoperitoneum

Pneumoperitoneum induced during laparoscopic surgery is another cause of iatrogenic raised IAP.

Insufflation pressure is usually kept at 10–15 mmHg. This pressure reflects the pressure in the non-dependent part of the peritoneal cavity. The pressure in the dependent part might be significantly higher owing to the weight of the splanchnic organs. Pneumoperitoneum gives similar symptoms as IAH or ACS, with respiratory and circulatory compromises, including reduced perfusion of the kidneys and splanchnic organs.

An increase in liver enzymes can be measured owing to compromised hepatic circulation. Diuresis usually decreases during the pneumoperitoneum and in infants may lead to transient anuria. Alterations in circulation and respiration are reversible and sustained effects are rarely seen if the pneumoperitoneum is only present for a short period of time.

IAP in the haematological patient

Haematological patients have several reasons to present with IAP. These are listed in Table 14.1.

Any other conditions leading to IAP?

IAP is recognized as playing a major role in many different pathological entities.

Table 14.1 Increased IAP in the haematological patient

Growth factor-induced capillary leak syndrome with concomitant large volume fluid resuscitation and third space sequestration

Chemotherapy-induced ileus, colonic pseudo-obstruction (Ogilvie's syndrome), mucositis or gastroenteritis

Sepsis and infectious complications aggravating intestinal and capillary permeability

Extramedullary haematopoiesis as seen with chronic myeloid leukaemia resulting in hepatosplenomegaly, chronic IAH and chronic (irreversible) pulmonary hypertension

The mechanisms of veno-occlusive disease seen after stem cell transplantation may be triggered by, or related to, increased IAP

Gastroenterology

ACS has been described in patients with toxic megacolon related to *Clostridium difficile*, gastroenteritis and perforated diverticuli. IAP can trigger (re)bleeding of oesophageal varices in patients with end-stage liver cirrhosis. This justifies the placement of a nasogastric tube to decompress the stomach after endoscopy.

ACS has been reported after colonoscopy.

Respiratory

Non-invasive ventilation with the head of the bed elevated to a 45° position has been linked to IAH because of entrapment of air in the bowel. ACS has been observed during tension pneumothorax. IAH has been reported in patients with chronic obstructive pulmonary disease.

Neurology

IAP has been reported to play a role in the malfunction of ventriculoperitoneal shunts in patients with hydrocephalus.

Cardiology

Prolonged bypass time during cardiac surgery has been linked to IAH. IAH is seen in chronic cardiac failure and is associated with worsening renal function. ACS can occur during extracorporeal life support, and IAP should be monitored. Devices to induce hypothermia after cardiac arrest use a closed loop with instillation of cold fluids into the peritoneal cavity. For safety reasons, these devices limit instillation of fluids based on IAP, which should be below 15 mmHg.

Gynaecology

Ovarian tumours such as mucous cystadenoma have been reported to cause ACS (see Figure 14.1).

Reconstructive surgery

IAH and ACS can occur after reconstructive surgery and affect viability of surgical flaps.

Orthopaedics

IAP has been associated with the activation of abdominal muscles in highly trained participants during sudden heavy loadings.

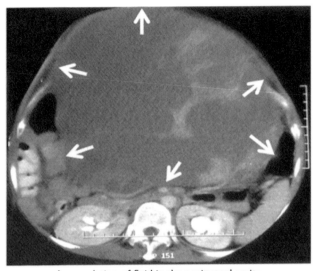

Accumulation of fluid in the peritoneal cavity
Arrows indicate increase in pressure
Kidneys and great vessels are compressed against the back wall.

Figure 14.1

Miscellaneous

ACS has been reported in scuba diving subjects, in a dog with babesiosis and in pigs with wheat bloating!

Key points

- Common clinical conditions (obesity) and procedures (laparoscopy, endoscopy, peritoneal dialysis) are associated with increased IAP and may produce similar symptoms to IAH or ACS.

- Some are not as severe as others and are usually rapidly reversible.

FURTHER READING

Chun R, Kirkpatrick AW. Intra-abdominal pressure, intra-abdominal hypertension, and pregnancy: a review. *Annals of Intensive Care* 2012; 2(Suppl. 1):S5.

De Keulenaer BL, De Backer A, Schepens DR *et al.* Abdominal compartment syndrome related to noninvasive ventilation. *Intensive Care Medicine* 2003; 29(7): 1177–81.

O'Rourke N, Kodali BS. Laparoscopic surgery during pregnancy. *Current Opinion in Anaesthesiology* 2006; 19(3): 254–9.

Schurig R, Gahl GM, Becker H *et al.* Hemodynamic studies in long-term peritoneal dialysis patients. *Artificial Organs* 1979; 3(3): 215–18.

Consequences of intra-abdominal hypertension: why to worry?

Chapter 15

Cardiovascular system and IAH

Introduction

Preload, contractility, afterload and oxygen transport are abnormal in the critically ill as a result of haemorrhage, fluid accumulation and direct cellular and organ injury. Inadequate resuscitation and failure to restore adequate cellular oxygen delivery through improved end-organ blood flow results in anaerobic metabolism, ischaemia and the development of multiple organ dysfunction syndrome.

Organ dysfunction observed during IAH and ACS is the result of pressure-mediated decreases in cardiac preload and contractility and increases in afterload. These phenomena compound the direct compression of organs.

Pathophysiology

Overall cardiovascular effects of IAH

Intrathoracic pressure rises during IAH. Up to 80% of IAP will be transmitted into the thorax. This leads to compression of the heart and reduction of end-diastolic volume.

Cardiac output is decreased because of the direct compression of vascular beds and activation of the renin–angiotensin–aldosterone pathway that causes decreased venous return and increased afterload. Mean arterial blood pressure may initially increase owing to redistribution of blood away from the abdominal cavity but will then return to normal or decrease.

Hypovolaemia and the application of PEEP will exacerbate the issue. Hypervolaemia will temporarily mask it.

A comprehensive list of IAH effects on haemodynamics is shown in Table 15.1.

Table 15.1 Cardiovascular effects of IAH – these effects will be exacerbated in cases of hypovolaemia, haemorrhage and with increased positive end-expiratory airway pressure

Diaphragm elevation and cardiac compression	↑
Pleural and intrathoracic pressure	↑
Difficult preload assessment	
Pulmonary artery occlusion pressure	↑
Central venous pressure	↑
Transmural filling pressure	↓ =
Intrathoracic blood volume	↓ =
Global end-diastolic blood volume	↓ =
Right ventricular end-diastolic volume	↓ =
Right, global and left ventricular ejection fraction	↓ =
Extravascular lung water	↑ =
Stroke volume variation	↑
Pulse pressure variation	↑
Systolic pressure variation	↑
Inferior vena caval flow	↓
Venous return	↓
Left ventricular compliance and contractility	↓

Table 15.1 (cont.)

Downward Starling curve shift to the right	
Cardiac output	↓
Systemic vascular resistance	↑
Mean arterial pressure	↑ ↓ =
Pulmonary artery pressure	↑
Pulmonary vascular resistance	↑
Heart rate	↑ =
Lower extremity hydrostatic venous pressure	↑
Venous stasis, oedema, ulcers	↑
Venous thrombosis	↑
Pulmonary embolism	↑
Mixed venous oxygen saturation	↓
Central venous oxygen saturation	↓
False negative passive leg raising test	↑
Functional haemodynamic thresholds for fluid responsiveness	↑

IAH and preload

In patients with IAH/ACS, elevated intrathoracic pressure decreases blood flow in the inferior vena cava and limits blood return in a pressure-dependent manner. Reduced venous return has the immediate effect of decreasing cardiac output because of decreased stroke volume.

The cephalad deviation of the diaphragm compresses the inferior vena cava as it passes through the diaphragm, further reducing venous return. This occurs with an IAP as low as 10 mmHg. It is also observed during laparoscopic surgery.

These changes in blood flow are likely to increase the risk of deep venous thrombosis.

IAH and contractility

Diaphragmatic elevation and increased intrathoracic pressure will affect cardiac contractility. Compression of the pulmonary parenchyma increases pulmonary artery pressure and pulmonary vascular resistance, and decreases left ventricular preload. The right ventricular afterload increases and the thin-walled right ventricle dilates, with concomitant increase in ventricular wall tension and myocardial oxygen demand resulting in a decrease in right ventricular ejection fraction.

The interventricular septum may bulge into the left ventricular chamber, impeding left ventricular filling and function with further decrease in cardiac output.

Right ventricular dysfunction can become severe in the presence of marked IAH, leading to significant reductions in left ventricular contractility.

Figure 15.1 represents the effects of IAP on left ventricular contractility.

IAH and afterload

Elevated intrathoracic pressure and IAH cause increased systemic vascular resistance through direct compression of the aorta and the great vessels. It also increases pulmonary vascular resistance by compressing the pulmonary parenchyma.

This explains why mean arterial pressure remains stable in the early stages of IAH/ACS despite the observed reductions in venous return and cardiac output.

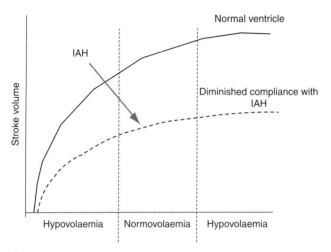

Figure 15.1

Implications for clinical practice

Filling pressures are inaccurate with IAH

Ventricular preload is directly related to the length of the myocardial muscle fibre at the end of the diastolic phase. Ideally, the clinician would measure the left ventricular end-diastolic volume to assess contractility precisely. This is not possible in practice.

Clinicians assume that the ventricular compliance is stable, and therefore a change in pressure is directly related to a change of volume (because Compliance = ΔVolume/ ΔPressure). Left ventricular end-diastolic pressure, left atrial pressure and pulmonary artery occlusion pressure are all used as surrogate estimates of intravascular volume.

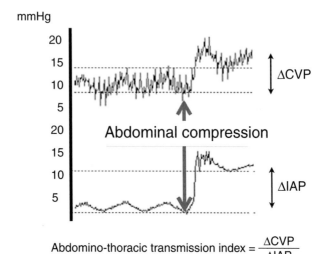

Abdomino-thoracic transmission index $= \dfrac{\Delta CVP}{\Delta IAP}$

Figure 15.2

These assumptions may prove wrong in the critically ill patient with IAH/ACS and could lead to inappropriate therapeutic decisions, resulting in organ failure. The abdominothoracic index of transmission can be calculated when both the difference in IAP and CVP are measured simultaneously (Figure 15.2).

Ventricular compliance is constantly changing in the critically ill, resulting in a variable relationship between pressure and volume. Changes in cardiac pressure no longer directly reflect changes in intravascular volume. The presence of IAH will decrease left ventricular compliance by rightward shift and flattening of the Frank–Starling curve (Figure 15.1).

The increased intrathoracic pressure associated with IAH has been demonstrated to increase central venous pressure measurements by an amount difficult to predict. This can be explained in part by central venous pressure being measured relative to atmospheric pressure when it is the sum of intravascular pressure and intrapleural pressure. It is beyond the scope of this book to try to explain these physiological differences, as many explanations are still only hypotheses.

Alternatives include measuring pressure during disconnection of the patient's airway. These may not, however, improve accuracy. The clinician should rely on trends and integration of IAP in his or her reasoning. Some clinicians will subtract half the IAP from the measured filling pressure.

What about volumetric monitoring?

The global ventricular end-diastolic volume (GEDV) is independent of the effects of changing ventricular compliance and increased intrathoracic pressure or IAP. Calculation of this parameter requires transpulmonary thermodilution measurements using devices such as the PiCCO (Pulsion Medical Systems, Munich, Germany).

Abdominal perfusion pressure (APP)

There is not a single 'critical' IAP that can guide clinical decisions in patients with IAH. While IAP is a major determinant of patient outcome during critical illness, the IAP that defines both IAH and ACS clearly varies from patient to

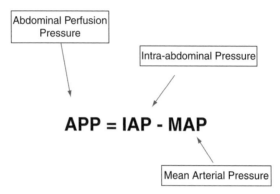

Figure 15.3

patient and within the same patient as the disease process evolves.

Analogous to cerebral perfusion pressure, the APP (see Figure 15.3) is a better endpoint for resuscitation in patients with IAH.

Maintaining the APP at 50–60 mmHg appears to improve survival in patients with IAH/ACS. Target APP values may be maintained through a balance of judicious fluid resuscitation and the use of vasoactive drugs.

Interactions between IAP, cardiac output and APP are shown in Figure 15.4.

IAP and responsiveness to fluid

An increase in IAP will result in a concomitant increase in stroke volume variation (SVV) and pulse pressure variation (PPV). This is explained by a change in aortic compliance and

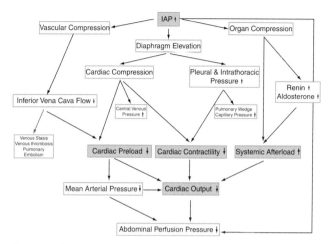

Figure 15.4

the increase in aortic transmural pressure induced by IAP (either via direct compression or increased vasomotor tone). Stroke volume variation and pulse pressure variation indices will be affected by the increased intrathoracic pressures and consequent changes in pleural pressure and chest wall elasticity. Many factors will render the interpretation complex, such as obesity, heart failure, pulmonary hypertension or pneumoperitoneum.

IAP will impair the venous return from the legs and mesenteric veins, and elevating the legs to test responsiveness may not be accurate. Raising the legs when the patient is sitting upright (to decrease the risk of ventilator-associated pneumonia) will increase IAP and result in a small amount of increased venous return from the legs but not from the

mesenteric veins. These effects will be different if the legs are
elevated from a supine or Trendelenburg position.

Key points

- Cardiovascular dysfunction and failure are common in
  IAH or ACS.
- Accurate assessment of preload, contractility and afterload
  is essential to restore end-organ perfusion and function.
- Pressure-based estimates of intravascular volume are
  erroneous with IAH/ACS.
- Transmural filling pressures and GEDV better reflect
  preload.
- Patients with IAH should be resuscitated to an APP
  >60 mmHg.

FURTHER READING

Cheatham ML, Malbrain ML. Cardiovascular implications
of abdominal compartment syndrome. *Acta Clinica Belgica
Supplement* 2007; 62(1): 98–112.

Cheatham ML, White MW, Sagraves SG, Johnson JL, Block EF.
Abdominal perfusion pressure: a superior parameter in the
assessment of intra-abdominal hypertension. *Journal of
Trauma* 2000; 49(4): 621–6; discussion 6–7.

Malbrain ML, de Laet I. Functional hemodynamics and
increased intra-abdominal pressure: same thresholds for
different conditions . . .? *Critical Care Medicine* 2009;
37(2): 781–3.

Chapter 16

Respiratory system and IAH

Introduction

IAP markedly affects the mechanical properties of the chest wall and, consequently, respiratory function. Altered mechanical properties of the chest wall impact on ventilation, influence the work of breathing, affect the interaction between respiratory muscles, hasten the development of respiratory failure and interfere with gas exchange.

The effects that IAH has on the respiratory system are listed in Table 16.1.

IAH and acute lung injury

The abdominal and thoracic compartments are separated by the diaphragm. It is estimated that 25–80% of IAP is transmitted to the intrathoracic compartment.

Patients with primary ACS will often develop a secondary acute lung injury. The major issue is the reduction of functional residual capacity and the increase in chest wall elasticity. IAH will increase airway pressures (peak and plateau pressures), dead space and shunt; it will decrease transpulmonary pressures, dynamic and static compliance. This will result in

Table 16.1 Pulmonary effects of IAH

Diaphragmatic elevation	↑
Intrathoracic pressure	↑
Pleural pressure	↑
Functional residual capacity	↓
All lung volumes	↓
Extrinsic compression lung parenchyma	↑
Auto-PEEP	↑
Compression atelectasis	↑
Peak airway pressure	↑
Mean airway pressure	↑
Plateau airway pressure	↑
Pulmonary vascular resistance	↑
Alveolar barotrauma	↑=
Alveolar volutrauma	↑=
Dynamic compliance	↓
Static respiratory system compliance	↓
Static chest wall compliance	↓
Static lung compliance	=
Upper inflection point on pressure–volume curve	↓
Lower inflection point on pressure–volume curve	↑
Hypercarbia – $PaCO_2$ retention	↑
PaO_2 and PaO_2/FiO_2	↓
Alveolar oxygen tension	↓
Oxygen transport	↓
Dead-space ventilation	↑
Intrapulmonary shunt	↑
Ventilation perfusion mismatch	↑
Ventilation diffusion mismatch	↑
Oxygen consumption	↑
Metabolic cost and work of breathing	↑
Alveolar oedema	↑
Extravascular lung water (EVLW)	↑=
Prolonged ventilation	

Table 16.1 (cont.)

Difficult weaning	
Activated lung neutrophils	↑
Pulmonary inflammatory infiltration	↑
Pulmonary infection rate	↑

increased $PaCO_2$ and decreased PaO_2, difficulties in ventilation and subsequent weaning.

IAH and ACS and their causes are associated with an inflammatory response that may trigger or contribute to an acute lung injury.

Paradoxically, IAH might in theory decrease the risk of acute lung injury as it decreases transpulmonary pressure for a set airway pressure, as it directly affects chest wall elastance and pleural pressure. This is offset by poor alveolar recruitment and shear stress at opening and closing of the alveoli.

IAH and lung distension

The increase in IAP is the most common cause of increased chest wall elastance in acute lung injury. Measuring IAP provides an excellent method for estimating altered chest wall mechanics without the need for measuring chest wall mechanics themselves. The IAP also influences the shape of the pressure–volume curve of the respiratory system, lung and chest wall. This is shown when comparing patients with acute lung injury with or without IAH (Figure 16.1).

In the presence of IAH, compliance decreases with tidal volume, suggesting alveolar overdistension. In ventilated

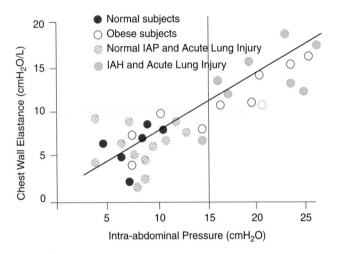

Figure 16.1

patients, abdominal compression results in decreased total respiratory system static compliance. The IAP value correlates with the lower inflection point or the best PEEP in ventilated patients with IAH. IAP plays a relevant role in determining changes in the chest wall mechanics and does affect lung distension during lung injury.

In the presence of IAH, higher opening pressures are needed to generate the same transpulmonary pressure to open the lung and higher PEEP levels are needed to prevent alveolar collapse.

IAH and pulmonary oedema

In a porcine model, it has been shown that the application of an IAP of 15 mmHg after oleic acid-induced lung injury resulted in an increase in pulmonary oedema. IAP of 30 mmHg causes high-grade atelectasis in the lower lobes of the lung. Increased IAP promotes lung neutrophil activation with increased pulmonary inflammatory infiltration and alveolar oedema. These changes can be explained by the increased cardiac filling pressures induced by the increased IAP and the decreased clearance of pulmonary oedema by lymphatics and capillaries.

IAP and mechanical ventilation

IAH decreases total respiratory system compliance by a decrease in chest wall compliance. Mechanical ventilation will usually increase IAP by 1–2 mmHg, and the application of positive end expiratory pressure (PEEP) will increase IAP by 1–2 mmHg.

An optimal PEEP value should be set to counteract the increase in IAP whilst avoiding overinflation of already well-aerated lung regions. Some clinicians advocate that the optimal PEEP in cmH_2O is equal to the IAP measured in mmHg.

Lung recruitment manoeuvres in the presence of IAH require higher opening pressures. Some clinicians advocate using a simple formula whereby they add half the value of the IAP in mmHg to the applied recruitment pressure expressed in cmH_2O.

During ventilation the body position will affect IAP. An obese patient in the upright position can develop ACS, and elevating the bed to 45° can increase the IAP by 5–15 mmHg.

The abdomen should hang freely during prone positioning.

During prone positioning care should be taken to avoid compression of the abdomen.

The reverse Trendelenburg position may improve respiratory mechanics; however, it can decrease splanchnic perfusion.

The reluctance to pharmacological muscle relaxation should be assessed against the beneficial effect on abdominal muscle tone, resulting in decrease in IAP and improvement of abdominal perfusion pressure. Muscle relaxation may be useful in patients with increased IAP during patient–ventilator asynchrony and help in reducing IAP.

IAP and pulmonary hypertension

IAH causes pulmonary hypertension via increased intrathoracic pressure, direct compression of the lung parenchyma and vessels and diminished left and right ventricular compliance.

Key points

- IAP affects chest wall mechanics and this has clinical relevance.
- IAP should be measured when assessing respiratory compliance.

FURTHER READING

Kirkpatrick AW, Pelosi P, De Waele JJ *et al*. Clinical review: Intra-abdominal hypertension: does it influence the physiology of prone ventilation? *Critical Care* 2010; 14(4): 232.

Pelosi P, Quintel M, Malbrain ML. Effect of intra-abdominal pressure on respiratory mechanics. *Acta Clinica Belgica Supplement* 2007; 62(1): 78–88.

Chapter 17

Renal system and IAH

Introduction

The decrease in cardiac output caused by IAH is an important contributing factor to acute kidney injury (AKI). A regional renal effect is also present, as demonstrated in animal studies where the ratio of renal artery flow to cardiac output decreased more than predicted with elevated IAP.

Both arterial and venous renal blood flow are decreased in the presence of IAH. This decreases the glomerular filtration rate. Renal venous hypertension is the most common cause of IAH-induced kidney injury. Renal veins are more prone to compression by IAP than renal arteries. Renal vascular resistance is increased more than systemic vascular resistance; this may be caused by the release of vasoactive mediators such as endothelin and/or hormones of the renin–angiotensin–aldosterone system.

The concept of renal perfusion pressure (MAP – IAP) may be used to explain decreased arterial renal blood flow in the presence of IAH, but correlation between renal arterial flow and renal perfusion pressure is weak.

Renal cortex microcirculatory flow is decreased in IAH models.

It is unknown if local renal parenchymal pressure plays a major role in the pathophysiology of AKI associated with IAH, but placement of ureteral stents does not prevent IAH-induced kidney injury, suggesting that ureteral obstruction is not a contributing factor. IAH-induced AKI is probably the result of multiple effects (Table 17.1).

Table 17.1 Renal effects of IAH

Renal parenchymal compression	↑
Renal perfusion pressure	↓
Filtration gradient	↓
Renal arterial blood flow	↓
Renal venous blood flow	↓
Renal vein compression	↑
Renal venous (back) pressure	↑
Tubular dysfunction	↑
Glomerular perfusion	↓
Glomerular filtration rate	↓
Diuresis (oliguria to anuria)	↓
Prerenal azotemia	↑
Urine sodium and chlorine	↑
Renal vascular resistance	↑
Corticomedullar shunting in renal plasma flow	↓
Effective renal plasma flow	↑
Compression of ureters	↑
Antidiuretic hormone	↑
Renin, angiotensin, aldosterone	↑
Sympathetic nervous system stimulation	↑
Arterial vasoconstriction	↑
Systemic hypertension in chronic IAH (obese)	↑
Adrenal blood flow	=

Incidence

AKI develops in approximately 30% of critically ill patients with IAH.

Critical IAP in relation to renal function

The relationship between IAP and renal function appears to be linear, with a greater impact at higher pressures. Clinically important renal dysfunction has been observed at IAP as low as 10–12 mmHg.

The impact of IAH-induced kidney failure

IAH is a strong independent risk factor for the development of AKI.

AKI is associated with high mortality rates. IAH and ACS are independent risk factors for organ dysfunction and mortality.

IAH-induced AKI often requires renal replacement therapy (RRT), leading to longer duration of stay in intensive care.

Implications for clinical management

Diagnosis of AKI in patients with IAH?

The pathophysiology behind the development of AKI during IAH is not well characterized. The first sign of IAH-induced AKI is oliguria. This occurs immediately when experimental IAH is induced.

In most critically ill patients, oliguria will be interpreted as prerenal in origin and justify an increase in fluid administration.

This leads to an increase in IAP and further deterioration of the kidney function. Considering IAH as a cause of AKI early in the diagnosis pathway is important as it affects the subsequent treatment.

Prevention of IAH-induced kidney injury?

Successful prevention strategies for AKI are based on fluid administration. Fluid resuscitation can be helpful in the presence of IAH if aiming to increase the abdominal perfusion pressure. However, positive fluid balance increases the IAP linearly and may therefore be detrimental. Other measures are required to avoid an increase in IAP.

The best prevention relies on IAP monitoring, and this should be done, preferably before or at least as soon as the kidneys become dysfunctional.

How do I treat the patient with IAH-induced AKI?

IAH is strongly correlated with the development of AKI. IAH occurs very frequently in critically ill patients (up to 70–80% in patients with septic shock). IAP must therefore be measured and lowered if elevated in critically ill patients with AKI.

Correcting positive fluid balance is critical and often requires limiting fluid administration. If this is not feasible or sufficient, a continuous infusion of loop diuretics may be effective. Whether diuresis can be increased by diuretics is uncertain. RRT is the ultimate treatment and ultrafiltration can rapidly remove large amounts of fluids and maintain fluid balance. If the patient develops ACS, appropriate measures should be taken without delay.

Peritoneal dialysis is not an option in patients with IAH since the added IAV will increase IAP, especially in patients with decreased abdominal compliance.

Both intermittent and continuous RRT have been used successfully to decrease IAP by removing excess fluids. From a practical point of view, continuous RRT provides minute-to-minute control of the fluid balance and this may be an advantage in very unstable critically ill patients.

Key points

- IAH is a frequent cause of AKI.
- The relationship between IAP and kidney function is dose-dependent.
- Clinically relevant kidney dysfunction may occur at IAP as low as 10–12 mmHg.
- The best way to prevent IAH-induced AKI is to prevent IAH.
- Fluid overload should be treated early and aggressively in patients with IAH and AKI.
- Peritoneal dialysis should be avoided in patients diagnosed with, or at risk of, IAH.

FURTHER READING

De Laet I, Malbrain ML, Jadoul JL, Rogiers P, Sugrue M. Renal implications of increased intra-abdominal pressure: are the kidneys the canary for abdominal hypertension? *Acta Clinica Belgica Supplement* 2007; (1): 119–30.

Dalfino L, Tullo L, Donadio I, Malcangi V, Brienza N. Intra-abdominal hypertension and acute renal failure in critically ill patients. *Intensive Care Medicine* 2008; 34: 707–13.

Shibagaki Y, Tai C, Nayak A, Wahba I. Intra-abdominal hypertension is an under-appreciated cause of acute renal failure. *Nephrology Dialysis Transplantation* 2006; 21: 3567–70.

Chapter 18

Central nervous system and IAH

Introduction

Abdominal decompression has been used successfully in the treatment of refractory intracranial hypertension.

In patients at risk of intracranial hypertension, care should be taken to avoid development of IAH. IAH must be treated in patients diagnosed with, or at risk of, developing intracranial hypertension.

Table 18.1 lists the physiological effects of IAH on the central nervous system.

How does IAH lead to intracranial hypertension?

IAP is transmitted to the thorax through upward displacement of the diaphragm. This leads to increased intrathoracic pressure. The abdominothoracic pressure transmission increases jugular pressure and decreases venous return from the brain.

Cerebrospinal fluid is pushed towards the spine to maintain a constant intracranial pressure (ICP). When compensation mechanisms are exhausted, such as in patients with cerebral oedema or brain trauma, the intracranial volume increases and the ICP rises.

Table 18.1 Central nervous system effects of IAH

Intracranial pressure	↑
Cerebral perfusion pressure	↓
Cerebral blood flow	↓
Jugular bulb saturation	↓
Cerebral venous outflow	↓
Cerebrovascular resistance	↑
Idiopathic intracranial hypertension in morbid obesity	
Pseudotumour cerebri in morbid obesity	
Neurological effects reversed after bariatric surgery or weight loss	
Neurological deterioration during laparoscopy	

The relationship between acute increases in IAP and ICP has been confirmed in several small series. Studies in pigs have confirmed that an IAH-induced increase in ICP is secondary to increased intrathoracic pressure as it does not occur after pleuropericardotomy and sternotomy.

Importance of the impact of IAH on ICP

ICP remains constant over a relatively wide range of intracranial volumes, as any increase in intracranial volume will be compensated by the drainage of cerebrospinal fluid through the foramen magnum. When these compensation mechanisms have been exhausted, any small increase in volume produces a marked increase in ICP.

If IAH occurs when ICP is already high (for example, after a trauma), any variation in IAP will impact on ICP.

Abdominal decompression has been used successfully to treat refractory intracranial hypertension in trauma patients.

Non-surgical techniques to decompress the abdomen, such as neuromuscular blockers and continuous negative abdominal pressure (CNAP), have also been successful in this context.

Conditions associated with increased IAP and ICP

ICP is increased during laparoscopy and this may be associated with increased incidence of postoperative nausea and vomiting.

Increases in IAP (such as with massive constipation) have been shown to cause ventriculoperitoneal (VP) shunt dysfunction and in some cases recurrent hydrocephalus.

Chronic increased IAP is thought to be an important factor in the development of idiopathic intracranial hypertension or pseudotumour cerebri in obese patients.

Implications for clinical management

Despite the absence of epidemiological studies on the relationship between IAP and ICP, the astute clinician will monitor IAP in all patients at risk of increased ICP. Neurological status should be frequently monitored in patients with IAH. Increased IAP should be considered as a possible 'extracranial' cause of intracranial hypertension in patients with abdominal trauma, even without overt craniocerebral lesions. In all patients with raised ICP, preventive measures should be taken to avoid any increase in IAP. In all patients with IAH, a possible association with raised ICP should be considered and preventive measures taken (e.g. head of bed elevation, avoid hypervolaemia, hypernatraemia and hyperthermia...).

Prevention of IAH-induced raised ICP

Measures to limit and control IAV increases should be instituted at an early stage. These include gastric suction if required, and frequent bedside ultrasounds to detect intraperitoneal fluids and prokinetics.

Restrictive abdominal bandages should be avoided in all patients.

Medical procedures increasing IAP (e.g. laparoscopy, colonoscopy, gastroscopy) should be avoided in patients with intracranial hypertension.

A major risk factor for IAH is massive fluid resuscitation. Control of the fluid balance is the cornerstone of IAH prevention. This may be complicated in patients with intracranial hypertension as fluid resuscitation is required to ensure adequate cerebral perfusion, especially in patients at risk of vasospasm (e.g. patients with subarachnoid bleeding).

There are no clear-cut answers to this clinical dilemma. One option is to use fluid administration to optimize cerebral perfusion in patients while monitoring IAP. A restrictive fluid regimen should be instituted when IAH develops.

Treatment of IAH when ICP is raised

Patients with intracranial hypertension need to be treated according to accepted international standards and guidelines.

IAP should be monitored in all patients with intracranial hypertension and risk factors for IAH.

Care should be taken to achieve euvolaemia. If the patient's intracranial hypertension is refractory to all treatment, decompression laparotomy should be considered.

Key points

- IAH leads to increased intrathoracic pressure, increased central venous pressure and decreased venous return from the brain.
- Increased IAP can lead to increased ICP in all patients.
- IAP monitoring should be performed in all patients with, or at risk of, developing intracranial hypertension.
- Prevention of IAH is essential in patients with intracranial hypertension.

FURTHER READING

Bloomfield GL, Ridings PC, Blocher CR, Marmarou A, Sugerman HJ. Effects of increased intra-abdominal pressure upon intracranial and cerebral perfusion pressure before and after volume expansion. *Journal of Trauma* 1996; 40(6): 936–41; discussion 41–3.

Bloomfield GL, Ridings PC, Blocher CR, Marmarou A, Sugerman HJ. A proposed relationship between increased intra-abdominal, intrathoracic, and intracranial pressure. *Critical Care Medicine* 1997; 25(3): 496–503.

Citerio G, Vascotto E, Villa F, Celotti S, Pesenti A. Induced abdominal compartment syndrome increases intracranial pressure in neurotrauma patients: a prospective study. *Critical Care Medicine* 2001; 29(7): 1466–71.

De Laet I, Citerio G, Malbrain ML. The influence of intraabdominal hypertension on the central nervous system: current insights and clinical recommendations, is it all in the head? *Acta Clinica Belgica Supplement* 2007; 1: 89–97.

Chapter 19

Other organs and IAH

The liver and IAH

The liver is particularly susceptible to injury in the presence of IAH. Hepatic cell function and liver perfusion are impaired even with an only moderately elevated IAP of 10 mmHg.

Acute liver failure, decompensated chronic liver disease and liver transplantation are frequently complicated by IAH.

Hepatic effects of IAH are summarized in Table 19.1.

The plasma disappearance rate for indocyanine green correlates with liver function, liver perfusion and with IAP. The function of cytochrome P450 will be altered by IAH/ACS and drugs should be adapted accordingly. Local haematoma formation within the capsule of the liver has an adverse effect on tissue perfusion and can cause a local hepatic compartment syndrome. Hepatic arterial flow and venous portal flow will decrease with IAH. This results in decreased lactate clearance, altered glucose metabolism and altered mitochondrial function.

Gastrointestinal function and IAH

IAH has profound effects on splanchnic organs with diminished perfusion and mucosal acidosis. The pathological

Table 19.1 Hepatic effects of IAH

Hepatic arterial flow	↓
Portal venous blood flow	↓
Portocollateral flow	↑
Lactate clearance	↓
Systemic lactate	↑
Glucose metabolism	↓
Serum glucose levels	↓ = ↑
Mitochondrial function	↓
Cytochrome P450 function	↓
Toxic metabolites medication	↓
Indocyanine green plasma disappearance rate	↓
Mucosal blood flow	↓
Intestinal mucosal perfusion	↓
Intramucosal pH (gastric tonometry)	↓
Regional CO_2	↑
Successful enteral feeding	↓
Gastric residuals	↑
Gastric dilatation	↑
Paralytic or mechanical ileus	↑
Intestinal permeability	↑
Intestinal oedema	↑
Bacterial translocation	↑
Multiple organ failure	↑
Visceral swelling	↑
IAP	↑
Bowel ischaemia	↑
Lactic acidosis	↑
Gastrointestinal ulcer (re)bleeding	↑
Variceal wall stress	↑
Variceal (re)bleeding	↑
Peritoneal adhesions	↑
Necrotizing enterocolitis (NEC) in children	↑

Table 19.2 Gastrointestinal effects of IAH

Abdominal perfusion pressure	↓
Superior mesenteric artery blood flow	↓
Coeliac blood flow	↓
Blood flow to intra-abdominal organs	↓
Mesenteric vein compression	↑
Abdominal venous hypertension	↑

changes are more pronounced after sequential insults of ischaemia–reperfusion and IAH.

IAH and ACS may be the second insult in the two hit phenomenon used to explain the multiple organ dysfunction syndrome. Clinical studies have demonstrated a temporal relationship between ACS and subsequent multiple organ failure. ACS provokes cytokine release and neutrophil migration, resulting in organ failure. ACS causes splanchnic hypoperfusion even in the absence of hypotension or decreased cardiac output.

Table 19.2 summarizes the effect of IAH on gastrointestinal function.

The pH measurement in the gastric mucosa has been shown to be inversely related to IAP. IAH can lead to intestinal oedema, ischaemia, bacterial translocation and, finally, multiple organ dysfunction. Maintenance of adequate perfusion pressure (APP >60-65 mmHg) is required to prevent these phenomena.

The abdominal wall and IAH

IAH has been shown to reduce abdominal wall blood flow by direct compression, leading to local ischaemia and oedema. This decreases abdominal wall compliance and exacerbates IAH.

Abdominal wall muscle and fascia ischaemia may contribute to the infectious and non-infectious wound complications (e.g. dehiscence, herniation, necrotizing fasciitis) seen in this patient population.

Table 19.3 lists the effects of IAH on the abdominal wall.

Endocrine function and IAH

Table 19.4 summarizes the effects of IAH on endocrine function.

Table 19.3 Effects of IAH on abdominal wall

Abdominal wall compliance	↓
Rectus sheath blood flow	↓
Abdominal wall ischaemia	↑
Abdominal wall oedema	↑
Wound complications (dehiscence, herniation, necrotizing fasciitis)	↑
Wound infections	↑
Incisional hernia	↑

Table 19.4 Effects of IAH on endocrine function

Antidiuretic hormone	↑
Renin, angiotensin, aldosterone	↑
Release proinflammatory cytokines (IL1b, TNFα, IL6)	↑
Relative adrenal insufficiency	=

Key points

- IAP is inversely correlated with indocyanine green plasma disappearance rate.
- IAP is inversely correlated with gastric mucosal pH.
- ACS may trigger bacterial translocation and MOF.
- ACS is the ARDS of the gut.

FURTHER READING

Diebel LN, Dulchavsky SA, Wilson RF. Effect of increased intra-abdominal pressure on mesenteric arterial and intestinal mucosal blood flow. *Journal of Trauma* 1992; 33(1): 45–8; discussion 8–9.

Diebel LN, Wilson RF, Dulchavsky SA, Saxe J. Effect of increased intra-abdominal pressure on hepatic arterial, portal venous, and hepatic microcirculatory blood flow. *Journal of Trauma* 1992; 33(2): 279–82; discussion 82–3.

Chapter 20

How to define gastrointestinal failure?

Introduction

Great variability exists in the terminology of gastrointestinal dysfunction in critical illness.

A list of types of gastrointestinal dysfunction is shown in Table 20.1.

Multiple organ dysfunction syndrome

The American College of Chest Physicians/Society of Critical Care Medicine (ACCP/SCCM) consensus document about the multiple organ dysfunction syndrome (MODS) defines an organ failure as a dichotomous event that is either present or absent, and an organ dysfunction as a continuum of physiological derangements. In ICU, the term gastrointestinal failure (GIF) seems more appropriate to describe severe dysfunction. 'Gastrointestinal dysfunction' is indeed used to describe a large variety of gastrointestinal symptoms (diarrhoea, vomiting) and diagnoses (gastroenteritis) that are not specific to the ICU patient. There is, however, no consensus about the term 'gastrointestinal failure'.

Table 20.1 Gastrointestinal dysfunctions

Gastrointestinal complications
Gastrointestinal haemorrhage
Non-haemorrhagic gastrointestinal complications
Gastrointestinal disturbances
Intestinal failure
Gut dysfunction
Upper digestive intolerance
Stress-related mucosal damage
Impaired gastroduodenal motility
Increased intestinal permeability
Inability to achieve an enteral feeding target

At its inception, the multiple organ failure (MOF) score evaluated seven organ systems: pulmonary, renal, hepatic, haematological, cardiovascular, gastrointestinal and the central nervous system. In this, GIF was defined as cholecystitis, stress ulcer, gastrointestinal haemorrhage, necrotic enterocolitis or pancreatitis and/or spontaneous perforation of the gallbladder. The revision of the score (15 years later) dropped GIF as its definition was not considered to be reliable.

The most recent revision of the MOF score includes GI dysfunction, again defined as ileus of more than 7 days or gastrointestinal bleeding requiring less than six blood products per 24 hours. GIF is defined as gastrointestinal bleeding requiring more than six blood products per 24 hours.

GIF has also been defined as the presence of mesenteric ischaemia, diverticulitis, pancreatitis, peptic ulcer disease or cholecystitis.

MODS can be defined as primary or secondary. Primary MODS results from a well defined insult in which organ dysfunction occurs early and can be directly attributable to the insult itself. An example of primary MODS is an organ dysfunction after trauma (e.g. pulmonary contusion, renal failure due to rhabdomyolysis, or the coagulopathy caused by multiple transfusions). In primary MODS, the participation of an abnormal and excessive host inflammatory response in both the onset and progression of the syndrome is not as clear as it is in secondary MODS. Secondary MODS develops as a consequence of a host response, and is identified within the context of systemic inflammatory response syndrome (SIRS). Secondary MODS usually evolves after a latent period following the inciting injury or event.

IAH as a marker of gastrointestinal dysfunction

The assignment of criteria to measure organ dysfunction should not occur *a priori*, but should result from an empirical process in which specific variables are tested against outcome.

Successful enteral feeding without any gastrointestinal symptoms usually suggests adequate digestive function. Unfortunately, measurements for failure or partial success of enteral feeding are not well defined and differ remarkably in the literature.

IAP and gastrointestinal symptoms both have an impact on patient outcome. IAP might be used as a surrogate for gastrointestinal function. On a physiological basis, it is probably correct to state that IAP influences gastrointestinal function and vice versa. IAH may be a cause or a result of GIF. The definite argument behind using IAP measurement is its objective and reproducible measurable value.

The combination of IAH and intolerance to enteral feeding into a scoring system shows a good correlation with mortality. Moreover, GIF is an important co-factor when integrated into the sequential organ failure (SOFA) score.

Implications for clinical practice

Any syndrome we aim to treat must first be defined. The failure to define GIF within MODS inevitably leads to the failure to treat the syndrome. We here propose definitions for gastrointestinal dysfunction/failure in ICU patients.

Gastrointestinal function is to absorb and digest food to extract nutrients, and expel the remaining matter. The gastrointestinal tract is responsible for ingestion, digestion, absorption and elimination. It is also a prominent part of the endocrine and immune systems.

Gastrointestinal dysfunction is a condition when the gastrointestinal tract is not able to perform digestion and absorption adequately to satisfy the nutrient and fluid requirements of the body. The condition is characterized by the acute occurrence of gastrointestinal symptoms associated with impaired digestion (e.g. vomiting, diarrhoea, etc.).

Gastrointestinal failure (GIF) represents the most severe form of gastrointestinal dysfunction. The condition is characterized by an acutely developed complete or near-complete loss of digestive function of the gastrointestinal system, where

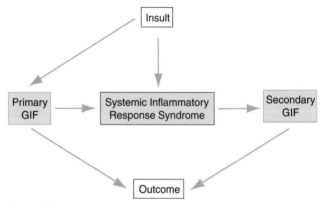

Figure 20.1

maintenance of homeostasis is not achievable without interventions.

Primary gastrointestinal dysfunction/failure is the direct result of an insult in which organ dysfunction occurs early (i.e. abdominal surgery).

Secondary gastrointestinal dysfunction/failure develops as the consequence of a host response in critical illness (i.e. gastrointestinal failure in a patient with pneumonia).

Figure 20.1 shows the different pathways leading to primary and secondary GIF.

Key points

- GIF is as important as other organ failures.
- Consensus in terminology and definitions has recently been finalized.

- GIF could be defined as a combination of success of enteral feeding and IAP.

FURTHER READING

Bone RC, Balk RA, Cerra FB *et al.* Definitions for sepsis and organ failure and guidelines for the use of innovative therapies in sepsis. The ACCP/SCCM Consensus Conference Committee. American College of Chest Physicians/Society of Critical Care Medicine. *Chest* 1992; 101: 1644–55.

Malbrain ML, Chiumello D, Pelosi P *et al.* Incidence and prognosis of intraabdominal hypertension in a mixed population of critically ill patients: A multiple-center epidemiological study. *Critical Care Medicine* 2005; 33(2): 315–22.

Reintam Blaser A, Malbrain ML, Starkopf J *et al.* Gastrointestinal function in intensive care patients: terminology, definitions and management. Recommendations of the ESICM Working Group on Abdominal Problems. *Intensive Care Medicine* 2012; 38(3): 384–94.

Reintam Blaser A, Poeze M, Malbrain ML *et al.* Gastrointestinal symptoms during the first week of intensive care are associated with poor outcome: a prospective multicentre study. *Intensive Care Medicine* 2013 (in press).

Chapter 21

Polycompartment syndromes

Introduction

A compartment syndrome arises when the increased pressure in a closed anatomic space threatens the viability of enclosed and surrounding tissues. Four major compartments are identified in the human body: the head, the chest, the abdomen and the extremities. An individual organ or a region with multiple organs can be affected in each of these compartments.

A compartment syndrome is not a disease and can have many causes.

Abdominal compartment syndrome

The abdomen can be considered as a closed box, like the skull. It has partially rigid sides (spine and pelvis) and partially flexible sides (abdominal wall and diaphragm) (Table 21.1).

The abdomen is filled with organs (small and large intestine, liver, kidneys, spleen) perfused by arterial, venous and capillary capacitance blood vessels (the mesenteric vessels) and filled with a fluid. This fluid only becomes apparent in pathological circumstances (ascites).

Table 21.1 Cranial and abdominal compartments

	Cranium	Abdomen
Organ(s)	Brain	Abdominal organs, gut
Fluid(s)	Cerebrospinal fluid	Ascites
Enclosure	Skull	Abdominal wall
Lesions	Tumour, haematoma	Blood, oedema, ascites, air, tumour
Pressure	ICP	IAP
Perfusion	Cerebral perfusion pressure	Abdominal perfusion pressure

The analogy to other compartments is not absolute, owing to the moveable diaphragm, the shifting costal arch, the contractions of the abdominal wall and the intestines that may be empty or filled with air, liquid or faecal matter.

APP is calculated as MAP minus IAP, and may be a better predictor of visceral perfusion and a potential endpoint for resuscitation by considering both arterial inflow and restrictions to venous outflow (see Chapters 2 and 5).

Other compartment syndromes

Hepatic compartment syndrome

Within the capsule of the liver, formation of a haematoma (e.g. caused by trauma or bleeding diathesis) may have an adverse effect on tissue perfusion, causing a local hepatic compartment syndrome.

The liver is susceptible to injury in the presence of elevated surrounding pressures, especially with IAH or ACS. Animal and human studies have shown impairment of hepatic cell function and liver perfusion even at slightly elevated IAP of 10 mmHg.

Acute liver failure, decompensated chronic liver disease and liver transplantation are frequently complicated by IAH and ACS. In these patients, the plasma disappearance rate for indocyanine green correlates with liver function/perfusion and with IAP.

Cytochrome P450 function may be altered in cases of IAH/ACS. IAH leads to decreased hepatic arterial flow, decreased venous portal flow and increased portocollateral circulation, causing physiological effects with decreased lactate clearance, altered glucose metabolism and altered mitochondrial function.

Renal compartment syndrome

IAH is associated with renal impairment (see Chapter 17). Elevated IAP significantly decreases renal artery blood flow and compresses the renal vein, leading to renal dysfunction and failure.

Oliguria develops at an IAP of 15 mmHg and anuria at 25 mmHg in the presence of normovolaemia and at lower levels of IAP in the patient with hypovolaemia or sepsis. Renal perfusion pressure and renal glomerular filtration rate have been proposed as key factors in the development of IAP-induced renal failure.

The reasons for these response have not been established and are likely to be multifactorial: reduced renal perfusion, reduced cardiac output and increased systemic vascular resistance, and alterations in humeral and neurogenic factors.

Within the capsule of the kidney itself, local haematoma formation (caused by trauma or bleeding diathesis) may have an adverse effect on tissue perfusion, causing a local renal compartment syndrome.

Pelvic compartment syndrome

In the pelvic region three major compartments (the gluteus medius and minimus compartment, the gluteus maximus compartment and the iliopsoas compartment) can be distinguished from the smaller compartment of the tensor fasciae latae muscles.

The pelvic compartment syndrome is rare. It is often associated with drugs and alcohol abuse, infections (necrotizing fasciitis) and the use of anticoagulant therapy. Its occurrence may eventually increase IAP and affect kidney function owing to bilateral ureteral obstruction and increased retroperitoneal pressure. Decompressive fasciotomy of the gluteal compartment is the treatment of choice.

Cardiac compartment syndrome

Cardiac tamponade is the result of a cardiac compartment syndrome. It occurs when there is accumulation of fluid or air in the pericardium that compresses cardiac cavities and impairs the pump function of the heart. This can be caused by trauma, haemorrhage, infection or tumour. As little as 250 mL of fluid can cause acute cardiac tamponade. A slow accumulation will lead to larger amounts of fluid.

A similar clinical symptomatology can occur when the intrathoracic pressure increases as a result of IAH. When the IAP rises above 10–12 mmHg, the cardiac output decreases because both preload and afterload are affected. Tachycardia will develop, mean arterial blood pressure will decrease and pulsus paradoxus may occur. Cardiovascular dysfunction and failure are common with IAH.

Hepatomegaly may develop in chronic or acute heart failure, and cause an increase in IAP.

Intracranial compartment syndrome

The intracranial content is confined within a rigid bony cage. Compensation mechanisms to respond to an increase in pressure include evacuation of cerebrospinal fluid. This will be impaired by IAH.

Moreover, treatment to increase blood pressure and maintain or improve brain perfusion may include fluid therapy; this may cause retroperitoneal and visceral oedema, ascites accumulation and IAH.

Intraorbital compartment syndrome

An acute orbital compartment syndrome is a rare but treatable complication of increased pressure within the confined orbital space. An intraorbital pressure greater than 30 mmHg may decrease ocular perfusion pressure. Clinical signs include eye pain, reduced ocular motility, diplopia and progressive visual deficit. Prompt treatment will prevent blindness.

The acute orbital compartment syndrome is different from an intraocular compartment syndrome as in glaucoma.

Limbs or extremity compartment syndrome

The extremity compartment syndrome is a condition in which the pressure within the closed muscle compartment increases to a level that reduces capillary blood perfusion. Permanent loss of function and muscular contracture may occur. The extremity compartment pressure can be measured via a needle connected to a fluid-filled pressure transducer system. Normal extremity compartment pressure should be less than 20 mmHg.

A crush injury with subsequent oedema and associated increased compartment pressure can be caused by the patient's own weight when rendered unconscious by poisoning, drug overdose, strenuous exercise or during prolonged anaesthesia. External causes of increased extremity compartment pressure are related to trauma with fractures (especially tibia) and tight plaster casts, muscle contusions, bleeding disorders, burns (with eschars), venous obstruction and arterial occlusion with postischaemic swelling.

The extremity compartment syndrome will result in muscle compression and rhabdomyolysis which can cause hypovolaemia, acute kidney injury and failure, coagulopathy, acute lung injury and shock. Fluid resuscitation can be used to counteract the deleterious effects of the extremity compartment syndrome, but it can also lead to increased oedema formation and further rise in compartmental pressures.

In cases of established extremity compartment syndrome, the only definitive treatment is decompressive fasciotomy and muscle debridement in case of necrosis.

Polycompartment syndrome

Initially the term multiple compartment syndrome was used in a study of 102 patients with increased intra-abdominal, intrathoracic and intracranial pressure after severe brain injury. It suggested that the different compartments within the body are not isolated and independent. The term polycompartment syndrome is used to stop confusion with multiple limb trauma with compartment syndrome justifying fasciotomy.

The polycompartment syndrome is a constellation of the physiological sequelae of increased compartment pressures in multiple compartments of the body. The abdomen plays a central role in the polycompartment syndrome and the effect of IAH on different organ systems within and outside the abdomen is well recognized.

The ultimate goal of treatment is not only to decrease the pressure within a compartment, but to improve organ function and to decrease mortality.

Key points

- Increased compartment pressures are independently associated with morbidity and mortality.
- The diagnosis relies largely on compartment pressure measurement.

- The effects of IAH on different organs within and outside the abdomen are well recognized.

FURTHER READING

Malbrain ML, Wilmer A. The polycompartment syndrome: towards an understanding of the interactions between different compartments! *Intensive Care Medicine* 2007; 33(11): 1869–72.

Malbrain MLNG, De laet I. A new concept: the polycompartment syndrome – Part 1. *International Journal of Intensive Care* 2008; Autumn: 19–24.

Malbrain MLNG, De laet I. A new concept: the polycompartment syndrome – Part 2. *International Journal of Intensive Care* 2009; Spring: 19–25.

Treatment

Chapter 22

Improvement of abdominal wall compliance

Decreased abdominal wall compliance leads to IAH

The relationship between IAV and IAP closely resembles the relationship between intracerebral volume and intracranial pressure (ICP).

In the cranium, any increase in intracranial volume will be compensated by the evacuation of cerebrospinal fluid through the foramen magnum at the base of the skull. When this compensation mechanism is exhausted, any small increase in volume produces a marked increase in ICP.

In the abdomen, fluids cannot be shifted easily into another anatomical space, but the abdominal wall is less rigid than the skull. The abdominal wall stretch will initially keep the IAP constant. This compensation is impaired when the compliance of the abdominal wall (C-abd) is decreased. In these cases, the increased IAV leads directly to increased IAP.

This will be impaired in some specific conditions associated with decreased C-abd such as abdominal eschars in burn patients, after abdominal wall reconstruction, the application of restrictive abdominal bandages or, more commonly, oedema of the abdominal wall after massive fluid resuscitation.

Measuring abdominal compliance

C-abd is not measured routinely in clinical practice.
Circumstances and signs pointing to decreased compliance can
be checked at the bedside.

   Decreased compliance should be suspected in all patients
receiving large amounts of resuscitation fluids, such as patients
with burns, severe acute pancreatitis, septic shock, severe trauma
and massive transfusion. If IAP is measured using a pressure
transducer and a pressure curve is recorded, it is possible to
record end-inspiratory and end-respiratory abdominal pressures
and calculate the ΔIAP (IAPei – IAPee) (note that the correct
IAP is measured at end-expiration). During inspiration, the
diaphragm and upper abdominal organs are displaced caudally,
making the craniocaudal length of the abdomen smaller. This is
almost fully compensated in normal circumstances by anterior
displacement of the muscular abdominal wall, leading to a very
small increase in abdominal pressure. In patients with decreased
C-abd, this compensation is impaired, meaning that abdominal
pressure will be increased markedly during inspiration.
Therefore, the ΔIAP (IAPei – IAPee) provides a measure of C-abd.
A low ΔIAP indicates a compliant abdominal wall, while a high
ΔIAP points to decreased compliance.

Preventing decreased C-abd

In patients at risk for IAH, all factors leading to decreased C-abd,
such as restrictive abdominal bandages or devices, should be
avoided. If patients are put in the prone position, careful

attention should be paid to adequate supports for the thorax and the pelvis to allow space for the abdomen to hang freely.

When an open abdomen treatment is used, surgeons should make sure that the temporary abdominal closure method used does not decrease C-abd. This can happen when negative pressure is inadequately applied, leading to a decrease in C-abd by retraction of the dressing.

Fluid balance will affect C-abd. Massive fluid resuscitation, especially using crystalloids, leads to oedema of the gut and the abdominal wall. This in turn decreases C-abd. Fine tuning fluid therapy to optimize tissue perfusion without causing complications of fluid overload is one of the greatest challenges in the care of patients with IAH.

Increasing abdominal wall compliance

An aggressive therapeutic strategy is warranted if C-abd is compromised.

All restrictive bandages or devices should be removed and constrictive eschars or scar tissues should be surgically released.

Neuromuscular blockers may be required but are associated with adverse effects, e.g. an increased incidence of ventilator-associated pneumonia and critical illness polyneuropathy. The balance between risk and benefit should be carefully considered.

Removal of excess fluids to improve compliance should be considered. This can be achieved using high dose loop diuretics in patients with normal or mildly impaired kidney function. Administration of albumin or other osmotically active compounds may be helpful to remove large amounts of fluids. Careful haemodynamic monitoring is essential during active fluid removal. In patients with advanced kidney injury, diuretics may no longer be sufficient to remove fluids. Ultrafiltration using either intermittent or continuous renal replacement therapy has been used successfully. Although positive fluid balance has been identified as an independent risk factor for mortality in several studies, it has never been demonstrated that active fluid removal strategies improve survival. Prevention of fluid overload through goal-directed and careful fluid resuscitation is recommended.

Key points

- Decreased C-abd is most frequently caused by excessive fluid resuscitation.
- Goal-directed fluid resuscitation is the first step in avoiding fluid overload.
- During open abdomen treatment, surgeons should pay attention to the effect of the TAC technique on C-abd.

FURTHER READING

Ball CG, Kirkpatrick AW, Karmali S *et al*. Tertiary abdominal compartment syndrome in the burn injured patient. *Journal of Trauma* 2006; 61: 1271–3.

De Laet I, Hoste E, Verholen E, De Waele JJ. The effect of neuromuscular blockers in patients with intra-abdominal hypertension. *Intensive Care Medicine* 2007; 33: 1811–14.

Chapter 23

Evacuation of intraluminal contents

How do intraluminal contents lead to IAH?

Intraluminal accumulation of fluid or gas is rarely a major contributor to IAH, but intestinal obstruction (usually complete) or colonic pseudo-obstruction (Ogilvie's disease) can cause a significant increase in intraluminal volume.

Similarly, ileus and accumulation of faeces in the large bowel may add to increased IAP. The latter is usually a slower, progressive increase.

Excessive use of sedatives and narcotics and electrolyte abnormalities may cause ileus.

Accumulation of air with gastric dilatation, as is sometimes observed during mask ventilation or with non-invasive ventilation, can cause an increase in IAP.

Ileus and IAH

Ileus is a common finding in critically ill patients, especially in patients with abdominal problems such as pancreatitis, peritonitis or abdominal trauma. It is also frequent in postoperative patients.

Numerous factors contributing to ileus are present in the ICU, including sedation and electrolyte disturbances, and some degree of ileus must be suspected in all patients with IAH.

Enteral feed

The use of enteral nutrition in patients with IAH should be considered. Adding extra volume to the abdomen may, however, increase IAP, and it may be preferable to decrease or even temporarily stop enteral nutrition in patients with rising IAP. Food intolerance is very frequent in patients with IAH, and attempts to initiate enteral nutrition should not be pursued aggressively.

Evacuation of intraluminal content

Nasogastric drainage can be a simple step to reduce IAP, especially in situations where it is obvious that gastric insufflation has occurred. Insertion of a colonic or rectal tube should be considered in case of ileus of the large bowel. The risk of perforation should be acknowledged and great care taken. Air and gas can more easily be removed when using tubes compared to blood, fluid or faeces.

Administration of prokinetic agents such as metoclopramide or erythromycin can help. In patients with Ogilvie's syndrome, slow IV administration of Prostigmin will result in a reduction of the intraluminal volume, and therefore IAP.

In some patients, accumulation of stools may cause or contribute to IAH, and enemas may be effective in reducing IAP.

When pharmacological measures and the above interventions are inadequate, endoscopic decompression should be considered. Dilatation or disorders at the level of the small bowel are often not easy to reach using nasogastric or rectal tubes, and the success rate of endoscopic procedures may be lower.

Surgical intervention

In some patients, IAH or ACS is the presenting symptom of partial or complete gastrointestinal obstruction requiring immediate surgery. Interventions aimed at reducing IAP should not defer a surgical intervention.

When haemodynamic instability is present, nasogastric aspiration is often adequate to reduce IAP temporarily and prepare the patient for surgery.

Open abdomen management is not always indicated once the obstruction and dilatation has been treated adequately.

When interventions to evacuate intraluminal contents fail, other measures, including decompressive laparotomy, should be considered.

Key points

- Various conditions lead to increased intraluminal fluid or gas content.
- Nasogastric suctioning is a safe and effective tool to reduce IAP.
- Patients with IAH may be fed enterally but feeding intolerance is a frequent problem.

FURTHER READING

Cheatham ML, Malbrain ML, Kirkpatrick A *et al.* Results from the International Conference of Experts on Intra-abdominal Hypertension and Abdominal Compartment Syndrome. II. Recommendations. *Intensive Care Medicine* 2007; 33(6): 951–62.

Chapter 24

Evacuation of abdominal fluid collections

Introduction

What are the causes of abdominal fluid collections leading to IAH?

The most common abdominal fluid collections are made of ascites and blood. The presence of blood in the peritoneal cavity can have several causes, but blunt or penetrating trauma are the most frequent. These conditions are usually treated with emergent laparotomy and the fluid collection is evacuated. IAH does not last long enough to cause significant organ damage. Shock and ischaemia–reperfusion are the most significant early contributors to organ damage. With the advent of non-operative management of solid organ injuries, accumulation of blood may lead to progressive IAH during the first days after injury. There is a significant risk of IAH and ACS after angiographic embolization of abdominal injuries.

Ascites may contribute to IAH, but often in a more insidious way. It may be present chronically in patients with primary liver disease and contribute to organ dysfunction if spontaneous bacterial peritonitis develops or acute on chronic liver failure develops. Increasing evidence shows that ascites plays a role in the development of the hepatorenal syndrome. In most ICU patients, ascites develops as an epiphenomenon of fluid resuscitation. These patients will have other signs of capillary leakage on clinical examination, including peripheral oedema and pleural effusion.

On rare occasions, fluid collections that are localized or contained within a solid organ may contribute to IAH. Massive pseudocysts in pancreatitis or cysts in benign or malignant tumours can present with signs compatible with ACS; organ dysfunction often develops more slowly and the fluid collections develop over days or weeks.

Although they can be easily accessed, retroperitoneal, diffuse fluid collections (e.g. in a context of acute pancreatitis) can contribute to IAH but are usually not amenable to evacuation.

What about more factors leading to IAH or ACS?

The cause of IAH or ACS is rarely isolated. Fluid collections may contribute to IAH but multiple other causes can be associated. Identifying the primary reason might be difficult. In patients with capillary leakage, fluid accumulation in the bowel wall or intra-abdominal organs and decreased compliance of the abdominal wall are often present. It is important to remember that intraperitoneal fluid collections are the only cause that can rapidly be treated in most patients.

Implications for clinical management

Do all fluid collections require drainage?

Percutaneous evacuation of fluid collections is mostly considered in the context of intraperitoneal collections. In rare occasions, retroperitoneal collections, abscesses or pseudocysts can be drained if large and easily accessible. It is difficult to quantify the volume of the fluid collection in the peritoneum, but small reductions in IAV can result in significant decreases in IAP.

How to drain abdominal fluid collections safely?

Percutaneous drainage (PCD) is generally a safe technique if adequate precautions are taken. In all patients, it is advisable to confirm the location of the fluid using ultrasound. The left and right iliac fossa are the most convenient locations for inserting a drain; the linea alba can be used. The safe location for drain insertion should be marked on the patient during the procedure and it is important to avoid the epigastric artery on the anterior abdominal wall. Preferably, the patient should have an empty bladder before the procedure. Coagulation disorders, when present, should be corrected. Areas of skin infection or abdominal burnt tissue should be avoided. Extra care should be taken in pregnant women or women with childbearing potential. When bowel dilatation also contributes to IAH, single evacuation is preferred owing to the risk of injury of the dilated bowel.

Which catheter should be used for draining fluid collections leading to IAH?

Several types of catheters can be used for draining abdominal fluid collections. The type of fluid will guide the choice, with small catheters for ascites and large bore for blood. Curved tip or straight tip catheters may be used. Catheters with multiple side holes decrease the risk of occlusion in patients who require long-term drainage.

If single drainage is considered adequate, regular paracentesis needles can be used; for prolonged drainage, these will usually be obstructed rapidly.

When is PCD to be avoided?

Patients having a clear indication for laparotomy should not be managed by PCD unless there is impending ACS. PCD can serve as a temporary measure to improve organ function prior to surgery. Bleeding disorders, pregnancy and bowel obstruction are relative contraindications to PCD. In the case of prior abdominal surgery, the risk of adhesions is significant, and the area of previous surgery should be avoided.

When does the patient need a (decompressive) laparotomy?

In most patients, the effect of PCD on lowering IAP is immediate. If the amount of fluid drained is lower than expected, the operator should check with ultrasound or turn the patient into the lateral decubitus position to redistribute the fluid. If there is no or inadequate effect, other measures, including decompressive laparotomy, should be considered. When there is a surgically treatable cause of IAH or ACS (such as abdominal sepsis), laparotomy should not be delayed.

Key points

- PCD will effectively decrease IAP, even if only a small amount of fluid is removed.
- PCD might improve organ function before surgery, but surgery should not be delayed because of PCD.

FURTHER READING

Cheatham ML, Safcsak K. Percutaneous catheter decompression in the treatment of elevated intraabdominal pressure. *Chest* 2011; 140(6): 1428–35.

Mullens W, Abrahams Z, Francis GS *et al.* Prompt reduction in intra-abdominal pressure following large-volume mechanical fluid removal improves renal insufficiency in refractory decompensated heart failure. *Journal of Cardiac Failure* 2008; 14(6): 508–14.

Parra MW, Al-Khayat H, Smith HG, Cheatham ML. Paracentesis for resuscitation-induced abdominal compartment syndrome: an alternative to decompressive laparotomy in the burn patient. *Journal of Trauma* 2006; 60(5): 1119–21.

Chapter 25

Correction of capillary leaks and fluid balance

Introduction

IAH is a frequent complication of diseases associated with a massive inflammatory response such as trauma, burns, pancreatitis or sepsis. This secondary IAH, defined by a sustained or repeated pathological elevation in IAP ≥12 mmHg, is caused by capillary leak with extravascular fluid overload, leading to abdominal wall oedema and accumulation of free intraperitoneal fluid.

Awareness of the importance of IAP and prevention of secondary IAH are essential in avoiding IAH-induced organ dysfunction. This requires very careful fluid management from the earliest stages of treatment up to resolution of the underlying disease.

How does systemic inflammation lead to (secondary) IAH?

All diseases associated with the systemic inflammatory response syndrome (SIRS) cause endothelial dysfunction with increased permeability of the capillary wall. This leads to leakage of fluids into the interstitial space (causing generalized

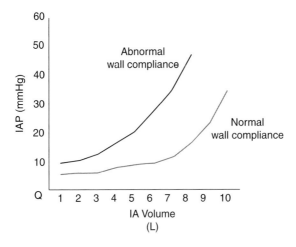

Figure 25.1

oedema) and later to accumulation of free fluid in the peritoneal cavity.

This increases IAV which in turn increases IAP. It leads to decreased abdominal wall compliance (C-abd) which increases the effect of added IAV on IAP (Figure 25.1).

The loss of fluids from the intravascular to the interstitial fluid compartment leads to intravascular hypovolaemia, which prompts further fluid resuscitation and ongoing oedema formation. Several studies have shown that fluid balance and IAP are correlated in a linear fashion.

Incidence

Secondary IAH is a frequent complication in many populations of critically ill or injured patients. It seems to be more frequent because of the recent emphasis placed on the importance of early aggressive fluid resuscitation.

IAH develops in around 30% of critically ill patients. Primary IAH is only slightly more prevalent than secondary IAH and mortality is higher for secondary IAH than for primary IAH.

Consequences of secondary IAH

IAH is a frequent cause of organ dysfunction and mortality in critically ill patients. The adverse effect of increased IAP on different organ systems seems to occur at different thresholds for different organs, but is usually dose-dependent (the higher the IAP, the more effect on organ function).

The kidney seems to be especially vulnerable to IAH-induced injury. This leads to decreased capability to clear fluids and, if not managed correctly, to fluid overload and aggravation of the problem.

IAH interferes with all 'traditional' haemodynamic monitoring tools, which makes evaluation of intravascular volume status and fluid responsiveness cumbersome. The detrimental effect of increased IAP on other organ systems is described in other chapters.

Implications for clinical management

How to prevent development of secondary IAH?

Many types of trauma or disease are associated with an increased risk for secondary IAH, but the common mechanism is usually capillary leak and abdominal wall oedema. The development of capillary leak and excessive fluid resuscitation should be prevented.

What are the possible interventions for capillary leak syndrome?

There is no specific therapy designed to abrogate capillary leak syndrome per se, but the clinician has several options available that may be utilized to minimize the expected sequelae.

Decreasing the amount of crystalloid given during resuscitation might make sense, and could be argued to be physiologically internally consistent. It is supported by some ARDSNet-related investigations. In these studies, patients managed with a 'restrictive' fluid management scheme fared equally well and, in some ways, better than those managed with a 'liberal' fluid management strategy.

Colloid fluid resuscitation offers an alternative approach to plasma volume expansion. Colloids are polydispersed, but generally have a three-dimensional size that impedes their extravasation across the capillary membrane. Many colloids are quite vast in size, and are often implicated in sepsis resuscitation as triggers for acute renal failure. However, smaller and less substituted colloids whose molecular weight and size still exceed the capillary leak pore size are now available. These products appear to be safer and just as efficacious with regard to plasma volume expansion as their larger, more substituted and older counterparts. Controversy surrounding the use of crystalloids or colloids still exists.

Utilizing biologically active colloids, including fresh frozen plasma, may be justified to address postinjury-associated coagulopathy and restore intravascular volume. Enhanced survival has been identified in military protocols using enhanced fresh frozen plasma to packed red blood cell ratios. It is unclear how much of the increased survival is related to more efficient perfusion correction and how much is because of reduced haemorrhage related to improved coagulation.

It is important to note that albumin is often utilized as part of resuscitation in diverse situations. Because of its small size, extravasation during capillary leak may be expected. However, as albumin has properties that include drug detoxification as well as transport, its influence on resuscitation in all but the brain-injured (in whom it appears injurious) remains unclear. Undoubtedly, this uncertainty will little influence albumin's use in the foreseeable future.

Judicious use of vasopressors to reduce precapillary arteriolar tone, increase cardiac performance and improve mean arterial pressure may reduce the absolute volume of resuscitation fluid required during shock management.

How is capillary leak prevented or diminished?

Causal treatment of the underlying condition or injury is the most important action to decrease the systemic inflammatory reaction that causes capillary leak syndrome.

Other anti-inflammatory therapies are being developed and may be considered in the future. In case of trauma or bleeding, early and aggressive control of the bleeding and correction of coagulopathy and acidosis is paramount. In patients with septic shock, immediate administration of antibiotics is equally important. Some disease states cannot be fully treated causally (e.g. severe acute pancreatitis, burns, . . .).

How are fluids used in the patient at risk for IAH?

Fluid resuscitation is essential in the treatment of most inflammatory states associated with shock. Studies have shown that early goal-directed therapy using fluids as a first step improves mortality rates in patients with septic shock.

However, as stated above, excessive fluid resuscitation in a patient with capillary leak also leads to oedema formation and accumulation of free fluid in the peritoneal cavity, which causes IAH. Studies have shown that supranormal resuscitation, e.g. in trauma, does not improve outcome and that positive fluid balance in critically ill patients is associated with increased mortality. Therefore, fluid resuscitation should be targeted to keep the patient's intravascular volume status and oxygen transport system adequate while avoiding over-resuscitation and leakage to the interstitial space and body cavities.

How is volume status and fluid responsiveness assessed in patients with IAH?

Studies have shown traditional measures of cardiac preload (central venous pressure (CVP) and pulmonary arterial occlusive pressure (PAOP)) to be useless in the presence of IAH because they are increased owing to cephalad displacement of the diaphragm and abdominothoracic pressure transmission.

Volumetric indices such as left ventricular end-diastolic volume index (LVEDV) or global end-diastolic volume index (GEDV) appear to be more reliable indicators of volume status. Stroke volume variation (SVV) and pulse pressure variation (PPV) have been advocated as parameters reflecting fluid responsiveness.

SVV and PPV are increased in patients with IAH and may not be reliable under these circumstances. On the other hand, the increase in SVV and PPV may indicate that patients with IAH do indeed respond favourably (at least initially) to fluid infusion, although, as explained above, one must bear in mind that fluid administration can further increase IAP.

Another simple bedside method to assess fluid responsiveness, autotranfusion through passive leg raising, may be unreliable in IAH, because the increased IAP impairs blood flow through the inferior vena cava and the autotransfused blood may not reach the right atrium.

The authors recommend the use of volumetric indices for assessment of volume status in patients with IAH. Fluid management should be aimed at keeping intravascular volume status in the lower euvolaemic range to preserve oxygen delivery and prevent development of IAH.

What fluids to use?

To minimize extravasation of fluid into the interstitial space it makes sense to use oncotic fluids that increase colloidal pressure within the blood capillaries, such as natural (albumin) or synthetic colloids (gelatins or starches).

Colloid use has raised some concerns regarding kidney function, coagulopathy and price. There is also the possibility (especially with low molecular weight molecules) that the colloids themselves may leak through the damaged endothelium and, because of their osmotic action, mobilize even more fluid into the interstitial space.

Studies in burn patients have shown that colloids can be used to minimize the amount of fluids administered, leading to a decreased incidence of IAH and organ dysfunction.

Another option to minimize the amount of fluid administration without causing hypovolaemia and organ failure is the use of hypertonic saline in certain conditions.

How is fluid overload associated with secondary IAH treated?

During the acute phase of their illness, patients will generally need large amounts of resuscitation fluids and, even if efforts have been made to limit fluid administration as much as possible, many patients will develop oedema and secondary IAH.

After the causal treatment for the underlying condition and the initial resuscitation have taken effect (e.g. antibiotics, source control, control of bleeding), care should be taken to remove excess fluids from the body as soon as possible to decrease IAP and improve organ function.

Diuretics (most often loop diuretics in continuous infusion) can be used to achieve fluid removal. However, secondary IAH is often associated with mild to severe kidney dysfunction, and patients may not respond to diuretic treatment. In these patients renal replacement therapy (RRT) with net ultrafiltration has been used successfully to remove excess fluids and lower IAP.

Since volume loading is well established as one of the few successful interventions to prevent acute kidney injury, it seems counterintuitive to aim for a distinctly negative fluid balance in critically ill patients with kidney dysfunction, but clinicians should be aware that IAH may be the cause of the acute kidney injury and treat it. Although there are few scientific data to support this, the authors feel that haemodynamic tolerance of fluid withdrawal can be assisted by using albumin 20% solution (either in 100 mL bolus administration or in continuous infusion) to increase colloid osmotic pressure immediately before and/or during diuretic or RRT treatment.

Key points

- Secondary IAH is a frequent complication in critically ill patients.
- Positive fluid balance and the development of secondary IAH are directly related.
- If the patient does develop secondary IAH, excess fluids should be removed using diuretics or ultrafiltration.

FURTHER READING

Cordemans C, De Laet I, Van Regenmortel N *et al.* Aiming for a negative fluid balance in patients with acute lung injury and increased intra-abdominal pressure: a pilot study looking at the effects of PAL-treatment. *Annals of Intensive Care* 2012; 2(Suppl. 1): S15.

Daugherty EL, Hongyan L, Taichman D, Hansen-Flaschen J, Fuchs BD. Abdominal compartment syndrome is common in medical intensive care unit patients receiving large-volume resuscitation. *Journal of Intensive Care Medicine* 2007; 22(5): 294–9.

Moore-Olufemi SD, Xue H, Allen SJ *et al.* Effects of primary and secondary intra-abdominal hypertension on mesenteric lymph flow: implications for the abdominal compartment syndrome. *Shock* 2005; 23(6): 571–5.

Chapter 26

Specific treatments for IAH and ACS

Introduction

Medical treatment of IAH includes improvement of the abdominal wall compliance (C-abd), removal of intraluminal contents, the evacuation of peri-intestinal and abdominal fluids, and the correction of capillary leak and positive fluid balance.

Alternative treatments for IAH and ACS have been described, but experience in humans is limited.

These include octreotide (OCT), continuous negative abdominal pressure (CNAP), traditional Chinese medicine and melatonin.

Octreotide in IAH

IAH has profound effects on splanchnic organs, causing diminished perfusion and mucosal acidosis. This sets the stage for multiple organ failure, with abdominal ischaemia–reperfusion as an important factor.

In animal models, it was found that OCT has protective effects on oxidative renal and pulmonary damage induced by increased IAP. A single intraperitoneal bolus of OCT was able to reverse the oxidant response in hepatic and intestinal tissues.

The use of OCT as a reperfusion injury-limiting agent cannot be recommended at present based on the current literature. Questions remain about safe dosing, frequency and timing.

CNAP devices

In animals, CNAP via a large poncho connected to a vacuum was able to reduce IAP significantly, and central venous, inferior vena caval and intracranial pressures.

In humans with pseudotumour cerebri, the ABSHELL™ (Figure 26.1) could rapidly reduce IAP from 19 to 12 mmHg, with concurrent decreases in intrapleural, central venous, jugular venous and cerebral vascular pressures.

In 30 patients in whom continuous negative extra-abdominal pressure (NEXAP) was applied (Figure 26.2), the average decrease in IAP was 4.5 mmHg.

The effects on the respiratory system have been more extensively studied in pigs. NEXAP reduced pleural pressures, resulting in higher transpulmonary pressures (and thus better lung volumes) and increased chest wall elastance.

When NEXAP is applied to the abdomen, the IAP will be reduced with minimal effects on mean arterial pressure and cardiac index.

Respiratory mechanics improve in patients with IAH. It is simple and easy to apply with minimal discomfort to the patient.

However, many questions remain unanswered and large scale experience in humans is lacking.

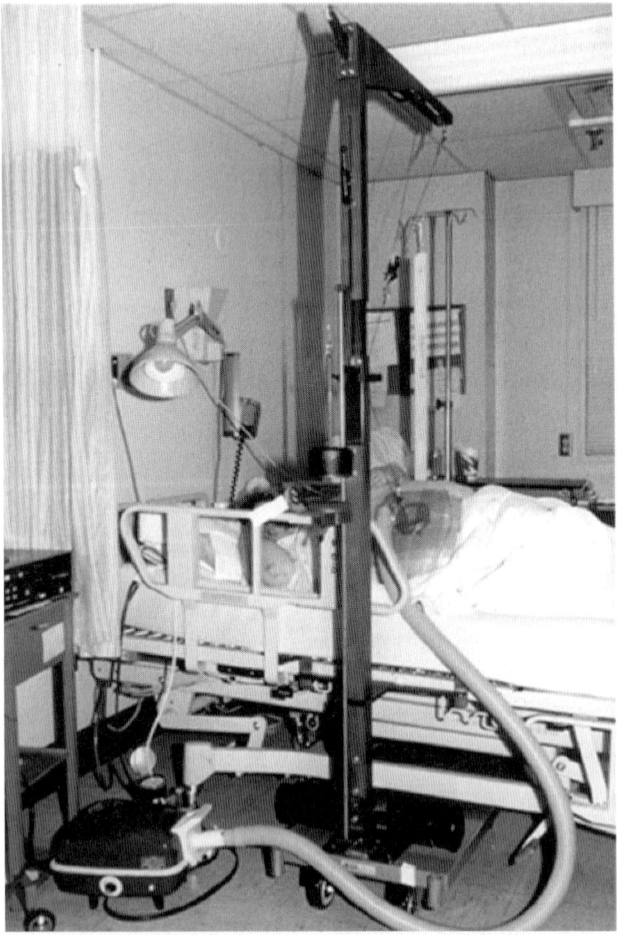

Figure 26.1 Patient in ABSHELL™ device with countertraction mechanism with patient rotated partially to the right. The tubing is seen from the ABSHELL™ to the vacuum pump on the floor by the patient's bed. (Reprinted with permission from Macmillan Publishers Ltd: *International Journal of Obesity* 2001).

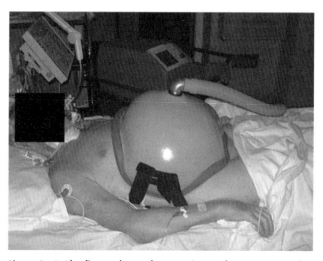

Figure 26.2 The figure shows the experimental apparatus used to generate negative extra-abdominal pressure. Reprinted with permission from Valenza F, Bottino N, Canavesi K *et al.* Intra-abdominal pressure may be decreased non-invasively by continuous negative extra-abdominal pressure (NEXAP). *Intensive Care Medicine* 2003; 29(11): 2063–7. ©2003 Springer Science and Business Media.

Traditional Chinese medicine

The effect of traditional Chinese medicines Da Cheng Qi Decoction and Glauber's salt were studied in combination with the standard treatment measures of severe acute pancreatitis, including parenteral nutrition, gastrointestinal decompression, continuous peripancreatic vascular pharmaceutical infusion, drug therapy and supportive measures.

Patients receiving traditional Chinese medicines had lower IAP at day 4 and 5, and mortality was reduced from 20% to 7%.

Da Cheng Qi Decoction is a traditional Chinese medicine that works as a prokinetic but unfortunately not much data in the western literature are available. Glauber's salt is used as an anti-tissue oedema agent but very limited data are available.

These findings might be explained by improvement of abdominal wall compliance via negative fluid balance (Glauber's salt) and evacuation of intraluminal contents via gastroprokinetics (Da Cheng Qi Decoction).

More trials, however, are warranted to recommend its use in acute severe pancreatitis.

Melatonin treatment

Studies have shown that melatonin has free radical scavenging properties and thus the ability to inhibit lipid peroxidation.

It has been demonstrated in the rat that reperfusion of decompressed tissue was associated with decreased levels of glutathione, increased malondialdehyde (MDA) levels (indicator of lipid peroxidation) and myeloperoxidase (MPO) activity. These levels were reversed when melatonin was given prior to decompression, confirming its protective effect on oxidative stress.

At the moment, however, we cannot recommend its current use in patients with IAH.

Nutrition

Malnutrition is a common finding in the critically ill patient and has been shown to be associated with increased morbidity (higher infection rate, delayed wound healing, prolonged mechanical ventilation, longer length of stay and duration of recovery) and mortality.

Even before admission to the ICU, critically ill patients are often in a catabolic state which will further deteriorate when haemodynamically unstable. High doses of supplemental vitamin C have been shown to reduce the incidence of secondary IAH and ACS in burn patients with over 20% total burn surface area.

The European Society for Clinical Nutrition and Metabolism (ESPEN) guidelines recommend starting enteral nutrition within 24 hours of ICU admission at 20–25 kcal/kg/day with at least 60% of the energy target reached within 3 days.

In patients with IAH, the intensivist faces a real challenge to deliver adequate enteral nutrition and, when there is failure to do this, it sets the stage for further systemic inflammation.

The four major risk factors to development of IAH and ACS are diminished abdominal wall compliance, increased intra-abdominal contents, capillary leak and fluid resuscitation, and, finally, abdominal collections of fluid, air or blood, which are often the cause of inadequate nutritional delivery. Taking into account the significant protein loss via an open abdomen makes this group of patients particularly prone to severe malnutrition.

Table 26.1 Actions needed to ensure proper delivery of nutrients

---

Insert gastric tube

Use of prokinetics at time of admission (*early!*)

Nurse patient at 30–45°

Use aggressively medical treatment options for IAH and ACS
(see Chapters 22–25)

Start early enteral nutrition and aim for 60% of 20–25 kcal/kg/day by day 3.
Aim for 25–30 kcal/kg/day after the acute phase (after 3 days)

In cases of an open abdomen, add 2 g of nitrogen per litre of abdominal fluid loss
to avoid further protein malnutrition

To deliver adequate nutrients to patients with IAH, we recommend the actions shown in Table 26.1.

Key points

- Several promising treatments, such as octreotide, melatonin and even Chinese medicines, cannot yet be recommended.
- CNAP improves respiratory mechanics in patients with IAH by reducing chest wall elastance.
- Open abdomen patients can safely be fed enterally.

FURTHER READING

Bloomfield G, Saggi B, Blocher C, Sugerman H. Physiologic effects of externally applied continuous negative abdominal pressure for intra-abdominal hypertension. *Journal of Trauma* 1999; 46(6): 1009–14; discussion 14–16.

Cheatham ML, Safcsak K, Brzezinski SJ *et al*. Nitrogen balance, protein loss, and the open abdomen[see comment]. *Critical Care Medicine* 2007; 35(1): 127–31.

Kacmaz A, Polat A, User Y *et al*. Octreotide improves reperfusion-induced oxidative injury in acute abdominal hypertension in rats. *Journal of Gastrointestinal Surgery* 2004; 8(1): 113–19.

Sener G, Kacmaz A, User Y *et al*. Melatonin ameliorates oxidative organ damage induced by acute intra-abdominal compartment syndrome in rats. *Journal of Pineal Research* 2003; 35(3): 163–8.

Valenza F, Bottino N, Canavesi K *et al*. Intra-abdominal pressure may be decreased non-invasively by continuous negative extra-abdominal pressure (NEXAP). *Intensive Care Medicine* 2003; 29(11): 2063–7.

Zhang MJ, Zhang GL, Yuan WB *et al*. Treatment of abdominal compartment syndrome in severe acute pancreatitis patients with traditional Chinese medicine. *World Journal of Gastroenterology* 2008; 14(22): 3574–8.

Chapter 27

Surgical treatment

Introduction

Once considered the only treatment for ACS, abdominal decompression remains the most effective treatment option in most patients.

The procedure rapidly decreases IAP, has an immediate effect on organ function and should not be reserved for surgical patients only.

Midline laparotomy is used most often, but minimally invasive therapy is a promising tool in the treatment of ACS.

Several pitfalls should be avoided, but surgical abdominal decompression has a low complication rate in experienced hands.

Can abdominal decompression treat ACS?

Abdominal decompression affects both the abdominal wall and IAV. Abdominal wall compliance (C-abd) will increase and the abdominal volume may be higher after decompression. During surgery, ascites or blood contributing to the IAV will be removed.

Numerous studies have demonstrated that decompression results in a significant decrease in IAP, although IAH with IAP between 12 and 20 mmHg often persists.

Surgical decompression will directly or indirectly affect markers of haemodynamic, respiratory and renal functions.

In patients with prolonged exposure to high IAP, irreversible damage to organs may have occurred. Other processes such as ischaemia/reperfusion, sepsis or burns may contribute to organ dysfunction, and these cannot be treated with abdominal decompression.

Surgical treatment is the most effective treatment for most cases of ACS.

Is surgical decompression safe?

Immediate morbidity and mortality related to the decompression are low when performed by an experienced surgical team.

Bleeding from a midline laparotomy is rare and usually attributable to coagulopathy.

Bleeding from other surgical sites can be a problem – haemostatic resuscitation, metabolic correction and rewarming to counter the coagulopathy are most important.

Early attempts (within the first week after decompression) to close the abdomen may appear counterintuitive for some, but are essential to avoid subsequent hernia.

Surgery is for all patients

Surgical decompression can be used both in surgical and medical patients. Various reports have reported successful abdominal decompression in a wide array of patients.

Surgeons may be reluctant to decompress an abdomen in a patient without any other indication for abdominal surgery.

On the other hand, surgical patients should not automatically be treated with surgical decompression.

For patients without a straightforward indication for abdominal exploration, surgery is reserved for those patients who fail medical treatment.

What surgical methods can be applied?

Most patients will require a full, midline laparotomy to decompress the abdomen adequately. It should be realized that IAP may not reach normal values after surgery.

Other incisions have been described for surgical decompression, including a bilateral subcostal incision (preferable in cases of severe acute pancreatitis as this makes later surgery easier), or lumbotomy to evacuate the retroperitoneum.

A less invasive technique is the subcutaneous linea alba fasciotomy (SLAF), a minimally invasive technique that incises the linea alba but leaves the skin closed, avoiding all problems related to open abdomen management and the need for a temporary abdominal closure (TAC) system. Although the decrease in IAP will be less than with full midline decompression, it may be sufficient in a considerable number of patients. A midline hernia will remain.

Burn patients form a separate category: although formal decompression may be indicated in some, abdominal eschars should be treated with escharotomy at an early stage.

Should abdominal decompression be the only cure for ACS?

This may be true for some patients.

Once ACS has developed, the chances of obtaining significant results with medical treatment decrease.

The best method to prevent ACS is to treat IAH, the prelude to ACS, using medical treatment options, or to prevent IAH from developing at all.

As IAH often develops after ICU admission, ICU treatment may contribute to the problem, with fluid, especially crystalloids, as the major contributor.

Implications for clinical management

When should surgical treatment be considered?

Surgical treatment should be considered in deteriorating patients with ACS who fail medical treatment, in patients with rapidly progressive organ failure and high IAP (>30–35 mmHg), and in patients with respiratory failure and progressive desaturation despite high levels of PEEP.

Can abdominal decompression be performed in the ICU?

In some instances theatre time may not be readily available, and bedside decompression can easily be performed.

When an additional intervention (e.g. bowel resection) is necessary or when the cause of ACS (e.g. haemorrhage) is not controlled, the surgical theatre is the preferred location.

What are the pitfalls when decompressing the abdomen in ACS?

These are outlined in Table 27.1.

Table 27.1 Surgical pitfalls of decompressing the abdomen

Mini-laparotomy incision	For adequate decompression, the laparotomy should be from the xiphoid down to the pubis. A mini-laparotomy results in a mini-decompression
Hypotension	A sudden increase in the abdominal vascular bed may result in a sudden drop of blood pressure, especially in hypovolaemic patients
Ischaemia–reperfusion	Decompression can result in a sharp rise in cytokines and contribute to hypotension
Bleeding	If the cause of ACS is intra-abdominal bleeding, the risk of bleeding increases when the IAP drops. Careful haemostasis is essential
Incomplete abdominal exploration	A surgically treatable cause of ACS and should be dealt with at the time of decompression. In patients with longstanding IAH or ACS, bowel viability should be evaluated
Reluctance to close the abdomen early	When IAP is low, organ dysfunction has subsided and abdominal closure is feasible, it should be pursued at the earliest opportunity

Is decompression an option when only IAH is present?

At present, surgical decompression is not recommended for patients with IAH.

Although case reports have been presented in which patients with IAH clearly benefited from surgical decompression, it is not clear if all medical treatment options had been previously exhausted.

Does every patient require TAC after decompressive laparotomy?

Most patients will need a TAC after decompression. Patients with a large IAV resected or drained (e.g. total colectomy in toxic megacolon or massive ascites that was not diagnosed before surgery) are possible exceptions to this rule.

Patients with preoperative IAH (but not ACS) and requiring abdominal surgery (e.g. for infection) may be closed primarily and avoid TAC.

Ischaemia–reperfusion is a significant problem after decompression and abdominal visceral oedema usually increases in the hours and days after surgery.

Key points

- Surgical decompression is the most effective treatment for ACS.
- Surgical treatment should be considered in patients who fail medical treatment and in unwell patients with high IAP >25 mmHg.

- Several methods for decompression are available; the exact options should be decided on an individual basis.
- Most patients will need some form of TAC.
- IAP monitoring should continue after decompression, and prevention of recurrent increase of IAP remains necessary.

FURTHER READING

De Waele JJ, Hoste EA, Malbrain ML. Decompressive laparotomy for abdominal compartment syndrome – a critical analysis. *Critical Care* 2006; 10(2): R51.

Leppaniemi AK, Hienonen PA, Siren JE *et al.* (2006) Treatment of abdominal compartment syndrome with subcutaneous anterior abdominal fasciotomy in severe acute pancreatitis. *World Journal of Surgery* 2006; 30(10): 1922–4.

Chapter 28

Open abdomen management and temporary abdominal closure

Introduction

Temporary abdominal closure (TAC) is a central part of open abdomen management.

Different techniques have been proposed, and often it is difficult to decide what is best for the individual patient.

Robust and effective options for TAC are available, but TAC should only be considered a temporary solution.

Formal fascial closure should be the goal, to be accomplished as soon as patient physiology allows.

Characteristics of an ideal TAC

Table 28.1 lists the characteristics of the ideal TAC.

Negative pressure therapy measures

Negative pressure therapy has been used for some time in the management of various types of wounds.

The earlier vacuum based techniques were self-made systems in which drains were placed on top of gauze in the wound, sealed with polyurethane dressing and connected to a negative pressure source of 20–25 cmH$_2$O.

Table 28.1 Characteristics of the ideal temporary abdominal closure technique

---

Universally available

Easy and fast to apply

Porous

Controls fluid loss

Prevents ACS

Leaves fascia and skin intact

Not reactive to bowel and organs

Easy to remove and to replace

Keeps peritoneal cavity sterile

Low cost

The application of higher pressures (100–150 mmHg) was introduced by the American company KCI in the Abdominal V.A.C. dressing, allowing the evacuation of excess abdominal fluid and keeping a constant tension on the fascia.

Implications for clinical management

What TAC technique is to be preferred?

No prospective study has demonstrated superiority of any of these techniques.

In a systematic review, mortality rates were lowest in patients treated with an artificial burr, V.A.C. or dynamic retention sutures. A study using historical controls found that the use of the V.A.C. device was associated with faster abdominal closure, lower duration of mechanical ventilation and decreased ICU/hospital length of stay.

The decision as to which TAC to use should be based on the available resources and experience. Techniques considered to be obsolete by some may prove valuable when resources are limited, or when not all commercial products are available.

More than one method is often available in a hospital, and the same patient may benefit from different techniques at different stages during the treatment.

ICU staff should be familiar with all of the techniques used by the surgical team.

Where to change the TAC

When significant problems are expected at changes of TAC (e.g. in patients recently operated for abdominal bleeding) or when formal surgical procedures such as bowel resection or anastomosis are required, the surgical theatre is the most appropriate location for TAC changes.

TAC can be changed at the bedside in the ICU provided all necessary tools and anaesthesia are available.

When to change the TAC

This largely depends on the underlying condition, but in most patients TAC changes can be safely performed every other day.

When intestinal ischaemia is suspected, more frequent procedures may be desirable. Frequent changes increase the risk of collateral damage to the gastrointestinal tract.

When to remove the TAC

TAC should be removed after the cause has been treated and IAH subsided. The abdomen should be closed as soon as possible.

Several methods aimed at progressive closure of the fascia have been developed to assist early closure; some of them are TAC techniques on their own; others can be used in combination with other TAC techniques.

Efforts should be aimed at early closure of the fascia. Experience shows that this is easier to accomplish in trauma patients compared to patients with abdominal sepsis.

Temporary abdominal closure techniques

Various methods for TAC are available, from basic, cheap and easy to more expensive and complex options.

Depending on the type of cover for the wound, and the control of fluid, three different categories can be identified.

Skin closure-only TAC

This is the most basic form of TAC. This can be done with sutures (usually a running suture) or with towel clips.

It is cheap, fast and universally available, but damages the skin and may be insufficient to prevent recurrent ACS. Fascial retraction is not prevented either.

Synthetic cover-only TAC

The abdominal wound is covered by a synthetic prosthesis. This can be a simple sheet cut out of a saline irrigation bag that is sutured to the fascia or the skin.

Silicone sheets can be used as.

Meshes of different material fall into this category. These can be absorbable or non-absorbable meshes that are sutured to the fascia. Each mesh has specific characteristics and disadvantages that fall beyond the scope of this book. A prosthesis can also be used to approximate the fascia progressively by reducing the size.

Negative pressure TAC

Self-made systems using drains connected to chest tube collectors (e.g. Vac-Pac) are the first step. The resulting pressure in the wound is low, but allows easy control of the fluid accumulation under the dressing and prevents uncontrolled spillage of fluid.

Higher negative pressures are applied in the true negative pressure TAC, such as the Abdominal V.A.C. dressing and the more recent ABThera™ (KCI) or Renasys (Smith & Nephew). This technique increases the negative pressure in the wound and in the abdominal cavity, resulting in active evacuation of ascites and postoperative fluid collections and reduction of bowel wall oedema. Adhesion between the bowel and the parietal peritoneum is prevented by a silicone sheet.

Fascial approximation techniques

These techniques are add-ons to one of the above techniques and are intended to approximate the fascial edges progressively.

Dynamic retention sutures are horizontal sutures placed in a catheter across the abdominal wound. These can be easily adapted when abdominal wall compliance improves.

The ABRA® Abdominal Wall Closure is a commercially available dynamic wound closure system that pulls the muscle planes together under low tension while leaving fascial margins intact.

Key points

- TAC techniques greatly simplify postoperative care for open abdomen patients.
- The choice of a TAC technique is based on experience, patient characteristics and available material.
- Three categories of TAC can be identified: skin closure-only TAC, synthetic cover-only TAC and negative pressure TAC.
- No prospective outcome studies have been performed comparing different TAC techniques.

FURTHER READING

Boele Van Hensbroek P, Wind J, Dijkgraaf MG, Busch OR, Carel Goslings J. Temporary closure of the open abdomen:

A systematic review on delayed primary fascial closure in patients with an open abdomen. *World Journal of Surgery* 2009; 33(2): 199–207.

Sugrue M, D'amours SK, Kolkman KA. Temporary abdominal closure. *Acta Clinica Belgica Supplement* 2007; 1: 210–14.

The future

Chapter 29

The future of IAH and ACS

It is difficult, if not impossible, to know what the future will bring, but it may be evident from the previous chapters that there are many things that we do not know about IAH and ACS.

There is a lot yet to learn about clinical management, and we can speculate that the future looks very different from the way in which we treat our patients today.

IAH is universally appreciated as a significant disease in severely ill patients

Although IAH and ACS are increasingly recognized as relevant in several types of patients, many physicians remain indifferent to this message. It must be acknowledged that IAH has only been rediscovered recently, and that insights into the pathophysiology are evolving. Studies including large numbers of patients are indeed lacking, as are intervention studies that could demonstrate a benefit.

High quality studies that include relevant patient numbers are urgently needed.

Pharmaceutical companies are unlikely to sponsor this kind of research as there are no specific pharmacological targets to prevent or treat the disease. We are left to rely on investigator-driven research in a disease with a complex pathophysiology occurring in various types of patients, which makes designing and conducting clinical studies extremely challenging.

Natural history of IAH shows that short-lived IAH can be tolerated by some patients

The adverse effects of IAH have been documented in animal models and confirmed in patients. The natural history of the disease is currently not clear.

Mortality is invariably high in most series of patients with ACS, but is not 100%.

What are the reasons that patients survive ACS without even considering the diagnosis of IAH or ACS? Is it because IAH is only an epiphenomenon in some patients, but more important as a cause of morbidity and mortality in others? Is it because patients are treated for IAH without physicians realizing it? Insights into the natural history of IAH are needed to answer these questions.

Continuous, hassle-free IAP measurement makes recognition of the problem easy

IAP measurement remains the cornerstone of IAH diagnosis and therapy. Although techniques have evolved greatly, transvesicular IAP measurement is most often discontinuous and requires manipulation by the nurse. Further improvements will make IAP measurement as simple as measuring routine haemodynamic parameters or pressures within other body cavities such as the skull.

This will also lower the threshold for measuring IAP and facilitate acceptance of IAP measurement in various settings.

Prevention is better than therapy

In recent years, the focus has shifted from ACS – the end-stage syndrome of prolonged exposure to elevated IAP – to IAH. Especially in the early stages, there seems to be a time window that allows preventive measures to be applied. This will be expedited by the development of simple tools for IAP measurement.

As clinical experience increases, true risk factors for IAH (not to be confused with conditions associated with IAH) will increasingly be recognized. This may vary across patient types: trauma patients may have different risk factors compared to septic shock patients or postoperative abdominal aneurysm surgery patients.

Medical management is the gold standard for IAH

Medical management of IAH is increasingly recognized as an important strategy to reduce IAP, and studies have shown that the need for decompressive laparotomy is reduced when it is applied. There are various targets for medical management, and we need to optimize the use of the medical management algorithm. Some strategies may work in some patients but not in others, and tailoring the therapy to the specific patient condition will allow a more straightforward and targeted application of these different tools. Also, diagnostics will increasingly be used to aid the selection of the appropriate intervention.

Decompressive laparotomy will no longer be a therapy for ACS

Abdominal decompression may be regarded as the sole therapy for ACS by some, but its importance will decrease as preventative strategies and medical management are more successful and open abdomen treatment is used in abdominal surgery in patients at risk for IAH.

Eventually, a laparotomy with the sole intent to decrease IAP will only be necessary in patients that have not been managed appropriately – either medically or surgically.

Open abdomen therapy is used selectively in the high-risk patient and for the shortest time possible

Leaving the abdomen open after a surgical procedure is to be avoided, yet in some patients this cannot be avoided. Proper patient selection will reduce repeated surgery and prolonged ICU and hospital stay in patients who do not benefit from the intervention.

When used, a strategy that is aimed at early abdominal closure is applied both by the surgeon and the intensivist, as prolonged open abdomen treatment is the most important risk factor for complications. This will enable the team to have all abdomens closed within 7 days.

Epidemiology

Considerable progress has been made over the past decade, but significant work still needs to be done. We must study and learn from the past and, at the same time, proactively 'invent' the future. As aptly described by Ivatury, IAH/ACS is '…a clinical entity that had been ignored for far too long … the mystery of IAH and ACS continues to unfold, transgressing the boundaries of acute and chronic illness and medical and surgical specialities'.

The future of IAH and ACS is in our hands, and the results of recent multicenter studies confirm the importance of IAH and ACS on patient outcome. For those who carry the mandate to further IAH/ACS research, the path ahead is clear.

Using available evidence, we must develop an IAH/ACS therapeutic bundle and apply it in a multicentred, prospective, outcome trial. It is time to pay attention to IAH/ACS clinically and to move forward with such a trial.

INDEX